GETTING CLEAR

EVERYTHING YOU NEED TO KNOW TO **CURE ACNE** QUICKLY, EASILY AND NATURALLY

JENNIFER SWINK, MAPC
MEDICAL AESTHETICAN

Getting Clear: **Everything You Need To Know To Cure Acne Quickly, Easily and Naturally by Jennifer Swink**

www.CelebritySkinScottsdale.com/gettingclear

Email: gettingclear@celebrityskinscottsdale.com

Printed in the United States of America

First Printing, 2018

ISBN 13: 978-0-692-90484-8

"For beautiful eyes, look for the good in others;

For beautiful lips, speak only words of kindness;

For poise, walk in the knowledge that you

never walk alone."

Audrey Hepburn

Thank you:

to my parents Robbie & Joseph for believing in me
and helping me fund this project,

to my children Jayden & Bella for their patience & understanding,

to my boyfriend Paul for his support and encouragement,

to my cousin Danielle for providing me a peaceful atmosphere and
serene place to stay and write,

to my best friend Sheri for the many late nights reading & editing,

and to all my clients, for inspiring and trusting me.

Table of Contents

Introduction

The idea of writing something to help people with their skin, health and happiness has been brewing since I became an aesthetician over eighteen years ago. Being a single mom with two teenagers and my own skin-care practice, I could not imagine where I would find the time and mental energy necessary to write a book about acne, but I knew I had to do it.

Early on in my career, I began to notice a trend in the types of facial treatments I was performing. Regardless of a client's gender, age or ethnicity, I would hear the same complaints over again. "I've tried everything to get rid of my acne and nothing works! I have seen the dermatologist, been on antibiotics, birth control, Spironolactone, Retin A, benzoyl peroxide and even tried Accutane! I have purchased expensive skin-care products and gotten all kinds of facials. I have stopped eating fried food entirely, and I still have ACNE!"

My clients were desperate to cure their acne. It did not matter what type of acne or how severe it was, all of them were suffering because of it. Many of them had lost their confidence and self-esteem as a result of dealing with chronic acne. They had also commonly spent a small fortune on painful procedures and products for any glimpse of hope to cure their acne.

Hearing their stories and not being able to provide any solid answers motivated me to learn everything I could about acne. I had the good fortune of working for a naturopathic doctor where I received priceless experience. I began to learn more about how health affects the aging process, our skin, and specifically acne. I combined this training with my professional experience, education in health psychology, and certification in nutrition and weight management, and implemented a more integrated approach to skin-care. Not only were my clients receiving professional skin-care treatments and products, they were also being educated on the effects of diet and lifestyle on their skin. I guided them toward the real solution—it is the impetus for this book. *Getting Clear: Everything You Need To Know To Cure Acne Quickly, Easily And Naturally.*

I modified how I had been doing my consultations, from basic "cover-your-ass" medical questions to spending more time listening and asking more questions. I allowed my clients to educate me. They taught me just as much about acne over the years as my education in skin-care had. I began to notice specific dietary and lifestyle patterns of behavior and treatment approaches among my clients that just did not work. Many clients reported similar symptoms and complaints of digestive issues, high stress levels, poor dietary habits or hormone imbalances. I used this information to connect the different variables that affect acne and why some treatments were more successful for certain people than for others.

I began helping my clients understand the gut/acne connection and how changes in their diet and lifestyle would improve their digestive health and clear their skin. Based on the information they provided, I sometimes recommended they seek out proper medical testing and treatment for a possible underlying health condition that may have been exacerbating their acne. I provided specific acne skin-care tips and advice learned from years in the biz as to what does and does not work. I also had to remind them that my clinical facials and cosmeceutical skin-care products, albeit pretty good, still were masking the underlying problem. I repeatedly reminded clients that having chronic acne is not due to having the wrong skin-care products. I had to tell them the hard truth. You cannot buy your way to clear skin.

I am sensitive to client finances and the costs involved with trying to keep "on top" of their acne. While my treatments and recommendations do help improve my client's acne, some clients are compromised, in my opinion, because they cannot afford to come in for a consultation monthly and sometimes weekly treatments. This book was written so that everyone from the projects to the penthouse can cure their acne with the program I have created.

Through countless hours of training and research, and with the support of my friends and family, I created *Getting Clear*. I am grateful for this opportunity to be of service to others in a way that improves not only their skin, but their quality of life. I feel a sense of joy and accomplishment with every person I have been able to help along the way. Having a client come in excited their acne is getting better is a priceless gift. Knowing I make a difference in peoples' lives fuels my passion and gives me purpose.

CHAPTER 1.
How We Got Here

Typically, chronic acne sufferers have tried it all with little to no long-term success. There are literally thousands of acne skin-care products and procedures that promise to clear your skin. Acne advice is everywhere from department stores, Internet, television, magazines, and your best friend, all claiming their way is the solution. You would think acne would be decreasing with all of this expert advice.

Instead, acne is on the rise globally. As more countries have become westernized, the incidence of acne has increased exponentially. The American Academy of Dermatology estimates 50 million Americans suffer from acne. Fifty percent of adult women and 25 percent of adult men have some form of acne. A study published by Foamix Pharmaceuticals (2017) reported there are 14 million physician visits per year for the treatment of acne. Acne is a multi-billion-dollar industry. The potential for revenue is virtually unlimited, and this has led to a marketing frenzy by opportunistic companies, at the expense of acne sufferers everywhere.

Acne is easier to cure than people might think. The problem is people are looking for the answers in the wrong places. Chronic acne is rarely eliminated permanently by topical solutions and prescription medication alone. It can be difficult to pinpoint the winning combination of acne products, and the right solution can differ from person to person. What is usually overlooked is how diet and lifestyle affect our body's balance and health that contribute to and exacerbate acne.

The interconnectedness of your body's systems is impossible to separate, so treating your acne with a singular approach rarely yields long-term success; sufferers experience an eventual resurgence in their acne regardless. Most of us do not want to waste our precious time and money on "maybes " for temporary results at best.

My goal as a professional is to help you *Get Clear* on what is causing your acne so you can cure it at its source. Accomplishing this will require an integrative approach that addresses all the underlying causes at the same time. The key to healing your acne is to attack it at root level, holistically, not solely with superficial solutions like topical products, or prescription medication like birth control pills or antibiotics.

INFLAMMATION, THE REAL CULPRIT

I am an aesthetician with decades of experience in my field. I have done extensive research on acne and how to treat it most effectively. Some of the information I found may shock you, and some of it may make perfect and logical sense. Either way, this information will help you get to the bottom of your acne once and for all.

The American Academy of Dermatology defines acne as a chronic, inflammatory skin condition. Chronic inflammation is also the cause of many diseases such as diabetes, coronary artery disease, Alzheimer's, rheumatoid arthritis and Crohn's disease, plus many more. It would then seem logical to assume reducing your inflammation will reduce your acne. Right? Interestingly enough, many of the conventional forms of treating acne such as antibiotics and topical retinoids can actually be pro-inflammatory, potentially compounding your acne.

The number of serious illnesses in the United States caused by chronic inflammation has skyrocketed and directly correlates to our eroding dietary intake over the last 50 years or so. I believe that the main causes of inflammation are diet and lifestyle. Diet includes the types of food and water you consume and medications you may be taking. Lifestyle addresses the amount and types of stress you experience, toxins to which you are exposed, and your sleep and exercise habits. These influence our overall health, both physical and mental. All of these factors directly impact your digestive health and consequently cause acne.

WHAT YOUR GUT CAN TELL YOU

One of the main areas our bodies take a major hit from diet and lifestyle is in our digestive health. An unhealthy gut is the real culprit in causing much of the inflammation we experience. What do I mean by "gut"? Your gut is part of the digestive system from mouth to anus, in other words, your gastrointestinal tract and all the organs along the way that help to keep us alive and healthy. We are a microbiome that consists mostly of bacterium that serve healthful roles in our guts. Your gut bugs, also known as intestinal flora, are just as vital to your health as your brain.

Diverse strains of good bacteria help digest food and absorb nutrients, help fight against bad bacteria and harmful viruses and serve to neutralize and detoxify harmful substances. These little friends produce and release vitamins, enzymes and neurotransmitters that keep our bodies happy and help us sleep well at night. The American Psychological Association reports ninety-five percent of serotonin is manufactured by specific bacteria in our gut. Gut bugs help to mitigate our stress and its effects on our hormonal system. Healthy, diverse intestinal flora reduces inflammation and its devastating effects on the body, one of which is acne.

In my research, I have learned that the corruption of our food supply has demolished our digestive health. The problem is what we're eating. Processed foods and the surplus of sugars, hybridized grains, gluten, dairy, genetically modified foods (GMO's), food additives, artificial sweeteners, chlorinated and fluoridated water, pesticides, plastics, parabens, aspirins, antibiotics and the physical stresses they put on our bodies cause massive amounts of inflammation. These foods (if you can call them that), not only kill off the quantity and diversity of your healthy flora, but also help multiply the growth of bad bacteria, yeast, parasites and viruses that wreak havoc on your gut's health and excrete endotoxins that cause inflammation. This can lead to a condition called "Leaky Gut Syndrome."

WHAT IS LEAKY GUT SYNDROME?

Leaky Gut Syndrome (intestinal hyperpermeability) occurs when junctions in the intestinal wall malfunction and allow unwanted allergens and substances (food particles, chemicals and other things) to leak into the bloodstream. This can cause a cascade of events, one of them being INFLAMMATION. Over time, if this condition persists, it can affect your skin and lead to various autoimmune disorders. Acne, vitiligo, psoriasis, rosacea, eczema, scleroderma and rashes are symptoms of leaky gut and possibly autoimmune disease.

If you have any diseases related to inflammation and/or an autoimmune disorder, you can safely assume you have leaky gut. If you have not been officially diagnosed with any medical conditions, start looking for these signs and symptoms of leaky gut before it turns into something much more serious than your acne.

- bowel issues – gas, bloating, chronic constipation, diarrhea or indigestion
- allergies – food sensitivities
- inflammatory skin conditions – acne, eczema, psoriasis, skin rashes, rosacea
- mood issues – depression and anxiety
- B12, magnesium, iron or zinc deficiency
- bladder infections
- chronic joint and muscle pain
- weight gain, for example, Syndrome X
- fatigue
- frequent colds.

NOTE: I strongly recommend you consult your doctor if you have any of these persisting symptoms. However, do not be surprised if your doctor is not familiar with leaky gut. Either way, these symptoms could be contributing to your acne.

CHAPTER 2.
Conventional Acne Methods

According to conventional medicine, there is no cure for acne. Maybe that is because many of the standard treatments do not work for everyone long term. **However, the fact that standard westernized medicine does not have the cure for acne does not mean there is no cure for acne.** Many physicians believe and tell their patients that the food they eat does not contribute to their acne. This is totally incorrect. For years doctors have been taught there is no connection between diet and acne. Unfortunately, nutritional training in medical school is very limited.

A survey in the <u>American Journal of Clinical Nutrition</u> (2010) found only 30 percent of medical schools require an actual nutrition course. This shocking fact, combined with the influence and profitable growth of the pharmaceutical industry, has dictated which acne treatments are prescribed. Topical and oral drugs are the only treatment options for acne dermatologists are qualified to offer.

Conventional medicine claims acne is genetic and caused by hormone imbalances. While it may be true your parents had acne and your hormones may be imbalanced, that doesn't necessarily equate to the cause. Fixed genes (you get what you get) are a popular notion, but we now know genes respond to everything we think and do. Our environment—like diet, stress levels, behavior and chemical pollutants—all affect the activity of our genes and our hormones. It is not our genes and hormones that cause acne; it is our diet and lifestyle that influence what our genes and hormones do or don't do.

Acne is commonly treated with various prescription medications, including Accutane, antibiotics, androgen blockers, oral birth control and topical skin products. It is not uncommon to be prescribed one or more of these treatments at the same time. In some cases, prescription medication may be necessary, but usually does not work long term because it does not address the root cause of the problem.

What's worse is that the overuse of antibiotics and other prescribed drugs have caused us to trade one set of problems (pimples) for another (undesirable side effects) and shift our focus away from healing acne at the source (diet and lifestyle influences).

Many of you may be reading this right now because you have tried some of these medications and still suffer from acne. Perhaps you are in the process of considering if any one of these conventional treatments is right for you. In acne grades III and IV, which is considered serious, it may be necessary to utilize the conventional approach short term. But, I recommend doing so only in conjunction with an integrative approach to ensure long-term acne-free success. Either way, I believe it is important for you to take your health into your own hands and educate yourself on the pros and cons of all of your treatment options. There is something to be said for self-advocating for your health.

ORAL MEDICATIONS

The typically prescribed treatments for acne are as follows:

- **Accutane** – (aka Roaccutane, Isotretinoin, Claravis, Myorisan) shrinks the sebum gland and reduces the oil it produces. This in turn reduces clogged pores, which reduces bacteria, which reduces acne. Accutane has an 80% success rate, yet a relapse rate as high as 47%.

  Various factors such as age, whether it is taken with or without food, dosage and duration of treatment, hormone imbalance and how well one metabolizes the drug affect an individual's success and relapse rate. The standard course of treatment is four to six months and is recommended be reserved for the most severe cases of acne.

My Recommendation: Only try Accutane as a last resort for serious stages of acne (cystic acne) and the onset of severe scarring.

NOTE: Accutane is known to have many dangerous side effects including, but not limited to, birth defects, bowel disease, depression, suicide, pancreatitis, erectile dysfunction and increased sensitivity to UV light which can cause hyperpigmentation, premature aging and skin cancer. Do not take Accutane if you're pregnant or trying to become pregnant.

- **Antibiotics** – Oral antibiotics (Bactrim, Vibramycin, Dorox) kill acne-causing bacteria inside the pores and reduce inflammation. While the use of oral antibiotics can be somewhat effective in reducing acne breakouts, typically what little results you see quickly disappear after discontinuing their use.

My Recommendation: Make sure to take probiotics while taking antibiotics to replenish good bacteria in place of all the bacteria being destroyed. Many of my clients have reported using antibiotics for months, even years to keep their breakouts to a minimum. DO NOT stay on antibiotics for long periods of time. Oral antibiotics should not be taken casually.

NOTE: Antibiotics are known to make skin more susceptible to sun damage and premature aging. They also can cause such side effects as yeast infections, digestive disorders and allergic reactions, to name a few. Since antibiotics kill both good and bad bacteria, they can upset microbiomes and promote inflammation. In the long run, they can make acne worse.

- **Birth Control Pills** – Birth Control Pills (BCPs) are used for acne in an attempt to lower or balance androgen (testosterone, DHT) levels with estrogen and progesterone. Assuming your acne is caused from elevated androgens, BCPs can be helpful in reducing acne breakouts. Be cautious because many BCPs can actually cause, or make, acne worse

My Recommendation: Make sure to check if your BCPs are indicated for acne. This includes Yasmine/Yaz, Ortho-Tri-Cyclen, Ortho-Cyclen, Desogen, Mircette and Estrostep.

NOTE: Some BCPs can cause hyper-pigmentation, so be sure to protect your skin in the sun. Be sure to investigate before using any birth-control method that contains hormones. Some IUDs contain hormones that could be contributing to your acne. BCPs can also create nutritional deficiencies, yeast overgrowth and the breakdown of intestinal lining.

- **Androgen Blockers** – Androgens are male sex hormones such as testosterone and DHT. Androgen blockers like Spironolactone, Propecia and Finasteride reduce acne breakouts, hair thinning and hair loss. In most cases, androgen blockers are used for treating acne in women only. Oral birth control and Spironolactone are often prescribed together because the combination works better at treating acne than either drug independently. Androgen blockers often take months to produce a reduction in acne breakouts and are not without side effects.

My Recommendation: A plant-based diet low in bad carbohydrates and sugars will lower or reduce high androgen levels naturally.

NOTE: Androgen blockers have serious side effects that include dehydration, diarrhea, dizziness, irregular menstrual periods, kidney problems and mood swings.

Propecia's potential side effects include sexual problems like impotence and abnormal ejaculation, swelling of hands/feet/breasts, dizziness, weakness and headaches.

TOPICAL MEDICATIONS

Topical medications, whether over the counter (OTC) or prescription, are helpful in reducing acne lesions. However, depending on the type and severity of acne, they usually are not enough to clear it long term. Most of the time, there is an underlying cause that needs to be addressed simultaneously for lasting results.

The most common types of topical medicines prescribed by doctors to treat acne are different creams or gels and include benzoyl peroxide, salicylic acid, topical antibiotics, steroids and retinoids. Some of these are described here:

- **Aczone** is a topical antibacterial and anti-inflammatory agent used to treat acne. Aczone seems to work better for women and when used in conjunction with a retinoid, rather than using either one independently. Side effects of Aczone include redness, dryness, itchiness and peeling of the area being treated. It is also possible that these side effects trigger an acne flare-up.

- **Retinoid** is a generic term used to identify topical forms of vitamin A (Retinoid/tretinoin/tazarotene/adapalene). Common brand-name prescriptions include Retin-A, Tazorac and Differin. Retinoids help to unclog pores, which reduce inflammatory lesions. They also help to reduce acne scarring and post-inflammatory hyperpigmentation. Topical retinoids and antibacterial agents complement one another and are often prescribed together. However, they can cause excessive side effects of redness, dryness, and peeling.

- **Benzoyl Peroxide** (BPO), both prescription and non-prescription, help to kill bacteria on the skin and dry up pimples. Common brand-name prescription BPOs are Benzaclin, Duac, Acanya, which combine Benzoyl Peroxide and an antibiotic. Epiduo is a prescription topical medication that combines Benzoyl Peroxide and Adapalene (retinoid). When used in the right dosage and skin-care routine, it can be helpful in reducing acne. Typically, OTC and prescription Benzoyl Peroxide can cause irritation, rash, itching and dryness. These side effects can trigger acne.

- **Antibiotics** can be offered in topical form and are designed to kill bacteria. The most common type of topical antibiotic are Clindamycin. Acanya, Benzaclin, and Duac. These are topical prescription medications that combine Clindamycin and Benzoyl Peroxide. Often, a combination of topical and oral medication is prescribed as a "go to" method of treating acne. Topical antibiotics may be combined with retinoids and benzoyl peroxide gels or lotions to kill bacteria, reduce oil production and unclog pores. Bacteria, over time, can become resistant to the antibiotics and alternative antibiotics may be prescribed.

When using prescription or OTC topical acne treatments, I usually recommend starting with the lowest dose, as with any product, and choose a gel or lotion form over a cream to avoid excessive dryness and overuse of moisturizer. If you decide to use a prescription retinoid, start with the lowest percentage of .025%. As your skin adjusts to the effects of the retinoid, you may be able to gradually increase the percentage if need be. To avoid dehydration, irritation, and inflammation, don't use multiple acne products on your skin. Be aware many of the ingredients in prescription and over-the-counter (OTC), topical acne solutions are full of inflammatory chemicals and pore-clogging ingredients. Confusing, right?

CHAPTER 3.
Integrative Acne Methods

Unconventional, alternative, holistic, integrative or preventative… slap any label on it that you want: Nutritional medicine and lifestyle modification are the most effective, long-lasting approaches for curing your acne. In my experience, westernized medicine has got it all backwards. Conventional acne treatments should be considered a secondary or adjunctive approach to treating acne, not the other way around. Diet and lifestyle changes should be the first line of defense against acne, and prescription medications should only be used when treating a more serious case of acne.

There is one thing both conventional and integrative medicine agree on: Acne is an inflammatory disease. Oil and inflammation are two factors that must be present to cause chronic breakouts. Oily skin can sometimes clog pores or cause blackheads, but without the inflammation part of the equation it does not cause papules, pustules, nodules or cysts.

We are genetically predisposed to have more or less oil in our skin. However, we do have control over the amount of inflammation we create in the body and similarly the skin. It may be hard to get chronic inflammation calmed down once it has started, but with dedication and a good plan, it is possible you can actively get it under control. Despite predisposition caused by genetics, it is possible to make skin oilier through the diet and lifestyle choices you make.

HEALING ACNE: AN INSIDE JOB

My overall recommendation for healing your acne is to start by reducing inflammation and healing your gut. Changing your dietary habits and lifestyle is the clearest path to creating a healthy digestive system and a clear face/body. In the interest of making positive and lasting changes, I recommend eliminating one or two specific food groups from your diet at a time or reducing your overall intake of these specific food groups. It will also be necessary to start eliminating toxins from your home and your body. Begin by eating fresh, organic, non-processed foods. Replace your household cleaning and personal-care items, one by one or all at once, with safer, non-toxic alternatives.

Stop assuming anything manufactured for your personal consumption or use is safe. I highly recommend doing research before you buy anything that you use around your home or goes on or into your body. This may sound daunting, but the goal is to educate and provide guidelines for eating and living in a perfect-world scenario. Understand your acne is a manifestation of internal imbalances usually caused by our choices and behaviors. Fix what's going on inside your body and the outside will follow suit.

The hardest part is getting started. If you want to clear your skin as quickly as possible, you must eliminate these foods outlined in the next section for a minimum of 90 days and 3 to 6 months is optimal if not indefinitely. It is possible once your gut has healed you may be able to re-introduce some of these food groups one-by-one in moderation to see if your gut or skin "reacts" or if it can tolerate it.

MODERN ISN'T ALWAYS BETTER

Technology is amazing, but when it comes to our food supply, modern isn't always better. In the interest of convenience, we all too often sacrifice good, healthy eating for quick, cheap alternatives like processed foods. Processed foods are any foods that are packaged in boxes, cans or bags. Examples are lunch meat, peanut butter, energy bars, ice cream, condiments, breads, breakfast cereals, juices, chips, crackers, pastries and pastas.

Processed foods, especially non-organic, typically contain harmful preservatives and food additives that are toxic. Pesticides, plastics and chemicals used in packaging contain hormone disruptors and gluten. Also, these foods are typically high on the glycemic index, which is the speed at which food increases blood sugar, and create insulin imbalances and inflammation.

Processed foods have the potential to include one, if not all, of these inflammation-causing acne-promoting ingredients such as high glycemic index carbohydrates, grains, gluten, soy, dairy, Omega-6 fatty acids, cooking oils, artificial food additives and environmental toxins.

Processed foods are a big part of the "westernized" or "american" diet. A westernized diet is characterized by a high intake of red meat, dairy, refined sugars, saturated fats, empty carbohydrates (junk food), processed and artificially sweetened foods, and salt. The westernized diet is low in fresh fruits, vegetables, whole grains, sea foods and poultry. Epidemiological evidence suggests that acne is considerably higher in westernized populations, indicating environment may influence the development of acne. This way of eating and the stress of Western life are triggers for acne. I believe both diet and lifestyle contribute to acne and the two are difficult to separate. Lifestyle affects food choices and food choices affect lifestyle

My Recommendation: Eat real food in its whole form whenever possible. Fruits (berries and citrus), vegetables and nuts provide good nutrients on the go. Always buy organic if you can.

DIETS THAT PROMOTE CLEAR SKIN

Following a plant-based eating plan rich in colorful vegetables and fruits, grass-fed/pasture-raised meats, nuts, seeds and spices is a solid dietary guideline. Plants are naturally anti-inflammatory and are full of all kinds of vital nutrients. Below is a list of anti-inflammatory, acne fighting dietary plans:

- **The Mediterranean Diet** – Includes fresh fruits, vegetables, plant-based proteins (beans and legumes), healthy fats (olive oil), fish, minimal dairy and red meat, whole grains and fresh herbs and spices.

  Many studies demonstrate people who eat Mediterranean have far fewer health problems than those on most other types of diets.

- **The Paleo Diet** – Based on foods eaten by early humans largely consisting of various meats, vegetables, nuts and berries. The Paleo diet allows for minimal dairy and excludes grains and processed foods.

My Recommendation: No diet that includes large amounts of meat could ever be considered anti-inflammatory. I would argue that it's not likely that our ancestors ate large amounts of animal protein on a regular basis when starvation was one of the biggest threats to their survival. Paleo is really plant-based, but allows for meat and minimal dairy. Therefore, a vegetarian could eat Paleo (a bit trickier) by just cutting out the meat and dairy. The main difference between the Mediterranean and Paleo is that the Paleo does not include grains. Decide which is a better plan for you based on your food goals.

- **The Whole30™ Diet** – A way of eating that eliminates certain food groups (sugar, grains, dairy and legumes) that could be having a negative impact on your health (acne) without you even realizing it. The Whole30™ helps to eliminate the most common blood sugar disrupting, gut-damaging, inflammatory food groups for 30 days. (refer to "Additional Resources").

Although people report significant improvements in all aspects of their health (weight loss, better sleep, more energy, etc), more serious or chronic health conditions, including digestive issues or acne, may take longer than 30 days to heal. This diet is like pressing the reset button on your health. The Whole 30™ diet changes your tastes, cravings and habits. This is the first place I recommend starting dietary-wise in clearing your acne. After completing the Whole30™ you may discover that one or more of the temporarily eliminated food groups will need to be permanently eliminated to remain acne free. Unfortunately, this is sometimes the case. It sucks, but having incurable acne is awful too. It will ultimately be your choice.

I actually did this diet for the first time 12 years ago, although it was not called the Whole30™ back then, after the naturopathic doctor I worked for suggested it to heal my "leaky gut". This was the first time I had heard this term. I was constantly getting sick with colds and bronchitis in spite of taking at least 20 supplements a day, eating predominately organic and exercising regularly.

On the outside, I appeared to have a very healthy diet and lifestyle. However, on the inside my leaky gut and chronic inflammation from the foods I was eating were depleting my immune system and causing me to catch every cold that came along. It never occurred to me that the food I was eating was what was making me sick. I assumed if I was allergic to or having sensitivity to a certain food I would get rashes, hives, nausea, or maybe diarrhea.

I learned these specific foods cause different health problems for different people, from typical allergy responses like itchy eyes, runny nose and rashes to weight gain, digestive issues, acne, and eczema—the list goes on and on—eventually turning into serious inflammatory and autoimmune disorders. The naturopath suggested I eat a diet free of processed foods, gluten/wheat, grains, beans, dairy and added sugar for at least 30 days.

Not only did I lose a few pounds, but I also stopped getting sick. I felt amazing. My skin looked fabulous. The whites of my eyes were white again. I was happier (less irritable or cranky). It forever changed my eating habits, and I never went back to eating quite the same again.

- **The GAPS Diet** – Similar to the Whole30™, the GAPS diet, also known as the Gut and Psychology Syndrome Diet, was created by Dr. Sidney Valentine to naturally treat chronic, inflammatory conditions in the digestive tract as a result of damaged gut lining. The GAPS protocol restricts all grains, processed carbohydrates, starchy vegetables and dairy to heal the gut lining, rebalance the immune system, and restore the gut's bacterial ecosystem. In addition to dietary guidelines, GAPS has a supplementation and detoxification protocol. Some of the recommended supplements include probiotics, essential fatty acids, digestive enzymes, vitamins and minerals. Light methods of detoxification and overall reduction of our exposure to toxins are also part of the dietary protocol (refer to " Additional Resources").

CHAPTER 4.
Foods that Contribute to Acne

TO GRAIN OR NOT TO GRAIN?

Grains such as wheat, barley, rye and spelt contain gluten that raises insulin levels, cause inflammation, digestive distress and damage your gut. They also contain phytic acid and lectins that create digestive problems and inflammation and prevent the absorption of vital nutrients and digestive enzymes. Whole grains are touted for having healthful fiber content, but there are other ways to get fiber, such as in fruits and vegetables.

David Perlmutter, M.D., author of *Grain Brain* wrote, "When I watch people devour gluten-laden carbohydrates it's like watching them pour themselves a cocktail of gasoline". Grains are naturally higher on the glycemic index (GI), a system that ranks different foods and their effect on blood sugar levels. Foods higher on the GI have more potential to negatively affect blood sugar and increase inflammation.

What about non-gluten grains like corn, rice and quinoa? To start, corn, rice and quinoa are high on the glycemic index. Thus, they are not optimal. Corn contains corn gluten, which is similar to wheat gluten and is also the most widely genetically modified food. Dr. Perlmutter refers to it as "Frankenfood". Many products labeled "gluten free" are made with corn or rice as a substitute. Also, farm animals which provide our meat and dairy, are fed corn-based diets. Corn consumption is often why individuals on gluten-free diets fail to heal because they are still ingesting gluten in another form.

What about rice? Rice is naturally gluten-free, assuming it is protected from gluten cross-contamination, free from flavored mixes containing gluten, or grain-based vinegars used to prepare sushi rice.

My Recommendation: Rice (especially brown rice) contains higher levels of arsenic, which is a toxic heavy metal linked to systemic inflammation and cancer. Rice is often used as a gluten-free substitute for adults and infants with allergies and gluten sensitivity. An excessive rice-based diet means more arsenic exposure. Read your labels carefully and choose brown, basmati rice from California, India, or Pakistan. These have less inorganic arsenic than other types. Buying organic rice will not reduce your exposure to arsenic; however, it will be free from pesticides.

What about quinoa? Quinoa is considered a safer gluten-free food alternative. Quinoa is not a grain, but actually a seed with favorable protein content. Seeds are typically harder to digest and contain lectins that can cause various digestive issues.

Quinoa is naturally gluten-free provided there is no cross-contamination. According to glutenfreesociety.org, a recent study found 41% of processed products randomly pulled from grocery shelves contain enough gluten to cause damage to those with gluten sensitivity (refer to "Additional Resources").

My Recommendation: Substitute grains with rice or quinoa in small amounts, provided you have investigated the food source, they are not cross-contaminated, and you do not already have allergies or gastric upset caused by these foods.

THE CASE AGAINST GLUTEN

What is gluten? Gluten is a protein found in many grains including wheat, rye and barley. Gluten acts as glue that helps foods maintain their shape. Because of its gumminess, it is used as a stabilizing agent in many products. Gluten is everywhere. It is in canned, baked, boxed, bottled and breaded foods. It is in beer, bacon, blue cheese, sauces, syrups, salad dressing, supplements, shampoos, cosmetics, condiments, cold cuts, creams and medications. If a product does not say "Gluten Free," you can assume it contains gluten. Of course gluten-free does not necessarily make the product healthy to eat.

So, what's the big deal with gluten? Gluten causes gut inflammation that can lead to serious health conditions over time. The proteins in wheat are like splinters digging into the lining of your gut causing inflammation and increasing intestinal permeability and leaky gut. Gluten also releases a protein called Zonulin that increases intestinal permeability by loosening the junctions between the cells in the gut wall to allow all kinds of "stuff" into the blood stream that shouldn't be there. Gluten can also affect female and adrenal hormone balance. Inflammation in your digestive tract can cause your adrenal glands to secrete cortisol (the stress hormone) that is directly associated with acne.

Gluten problems are not restricted to people with Celiac Disease. Gluten sensitivity or intolerance is a condition that causes a person to react after ingesting gluten. Symptoms vary widely and the degree to which they occur is different from person to person. Many times, side effects and symptoms are not associated with gluten consumption, or the effects go unnoticed until they manifest in more serious health issues.

Symptoms include gastrointestinal problems, joint pain, fatigue, neurological symptoms, chronic nutritional deficiencies, migraine, depression and skin problems like **acne**.

My Recommendation: It is my opinion that everyone is negatively impacted by the consumption of gluten regardless of whether they have known gluten sensitivities or not. I believe this an essential factor in the development of acne, and even worse, auto-immune disease. If you want confirmation, you can take standard gluten-sensitivity tests. Be aware these tests do not include all of the types of gluten used in the foods we consume.

THE EVILS OF SUGAR IN ALL ITS FORMS

There are 61 different names for sugar. Agave nectar, honey, cane sugar, corn syrup, dextrose, fructose, sucrose and fruit juice are a few of the more commonly recognized ones (refer to "Additional Resources").

A high intake of refined sugar and empty carbohydrates (sugars) negatively affect the hormone insulin, causing an increase in oil production and inflammation, which are both linked to acne. Artificial sweeteners, like aspartame, saccharin, Stevia and Sucralose, cause blood sugar spikes, raise insulin levels and alter the balance of your gut bacteria, causing inflammation, hormone disruption and potentially acne. Sugar also causes digestive problems by fueling the growth of bad bacteria, yeast and candida, creating an ideal environment for acne to occur.

My Recommendation: If you need something sweet, go for fruits lower in sugar content such as blueberries, blackberries, raspberries, strawberries, lemons, limes and grapefruit.

SOY CONFUSION

Most of us are consuming large amounts of soy without knowing it. Soy has been promoted as healthy, when in fact, it is not. Soy is a cheap filler and is commonly found in baked goods, candy, cereal, deli meats, nutrition bars, condiments, imitation dairy foods, infant formula, protein powders, sauces, and smoothies. The list is endless (refer to "Additional Resources").

Soy is one of the most prevalent food allergies. Soy reduces absorption of nutrients and can increase inflammation in the body. Inflammation, as you already know, increases the risk for acne. Soy contains phytoestrogens that can disrupt hormones that affect thyroid and estrogen levels. Consequently, when the ratio of estrogen and thyroid hormones to other hormones become out of balance, they can promote acne.

My Recommendation: Avoid soy. If you must consume soy, choose fermented soy. Tempeh and Miso are types of soy that have some health benefits, but I still only recommend eating these in moderation, if at all.

DAIRY, DAIRY QUITE CONTRARY

Although some people seem to tolerate dairy, we are not really meant to ingest it. It raises insulin levels, promotes excess estrogen in the blood and contains androgenic properties (hormones). High levels of androgens increase oil production that can trigger acne. Fat-free, low-fat, 1% or 2% dairy products are even worse than full-fat dairy, because once the fat is removed, the ratio of sugar increases and disrupts insulin levels. Also, dairy products, unless otherwise labeled, contain hormones and antibiotics that can disrupt your hormone balance and gut bacteria, increasing your risk for acne.

My Recommendation: If you are following a Paleo eating plan that allows for some dairy, it will still be a good idea to avoid dairy for at least three to four months while healing your gut and clearing your acne. If you decide to reintroduce dairy, make sure it is organic and does not contain antibiotics or hormones. Choose raw or unpasteurized full-fat dairy or goat milk/cheese. Although raw dairy is controversial, it is easier to digest.

PROTEIN POWDER OR PACKAGED PIMPLES?

With the rise of every fitness craze, you can bet not far behind is the nutrition plan that brings more convenience "foods" to be aware or leery of. Protein powders, shakes, and bars are very popular exercise supplements that are full of acne- promoting ingredients and fillers. It would be better to avoid protein supplements altogether and eat your protein instead. However, if you must drink it, choose one that is low on the glycemic index and make sure it is a plant-based protein powder free of dairy, wheat, gluten, soy, fructose, artificial colors, and artificial sweeteners.

CLARIFICATION ON COOKING OILS

Our bodies require a balanced ratio of Omega-6 to Omega-3 fatty acids. The westernized diet contains excessive amounts of Omega-6 fatty acids and is deficient in Omega-3 fatty acids. Canola, cottonseed, vegetable, sunflower, soybean and corn oils are common cooking oils that are high in Omega-6 fatty acids. These Omega-6 fatty acids are also commonly found in processed foods and fed to farm animals that wind up in the meals we consume. High levels of Omega-6 fatty acids are known precursors to inflammation, and inflammation can trigger acne.

My Recommendation: Avoid using the previously mentioned vegetable oils. Organic extra-virgin cold-pressed olive oil has a more balanced ratio of Omega-3 to Omega-6 fatty acids. Olive oil is best used for low-temp cooking, salad dressings and sauces. Coconut oil does not contain Omega-3 or Omega-6 fatty acids and is a great alternative cooking oil. Raw, organic cold-pressed coconut oil is especially good for cooking with high temperatures. Look for grass-fed beef and pasture-raised chicken and eggs to avoid consuming excessive amounts of Omega-6.

DON'T TAKE AWAY MY ALCOHOL

Alcohol is a triple threat. It damages your gut lining, breaks down to sugar quickly and dehydrates your body, all causing inflammation, hormone disruption and potentially acne. For these reasons, it's best to eliminate most alcohol completely. Certain alcohols are worse than others because of their high sugar content or because they contain grains and gluten. The Celiac Disease Foundation states that distilled alcohol does not contain any harmful gluten peptides because the gluten peptide is too large to carry over in the distillation process.

My Recommendation: If you choose to drink alcohol, only do so in strict moderation or occasionally. According to the

"Dietary Guidelines for Americans 2015-2020", established by the Department of Health and Human Services and U.S. Department of Agriculture, moderate drinking is up to one drink per day for women and up to two drinks per day for men.

Select gluten-free, grain-free liquors like potato-based or grape-based vodkas, tequila (100% agave only) or red wine. Avoid whiskey (bourbon), gin, vodka made from grains, beer, premixed sugary cocktails and white wine. It is important to drink the proper amount of water (based on weight) **before** beginning to drink alcohol. Consume a full 8 ounces of water in between each alcoholic drink to avoid dehydration.

YOUR DAILY DOSE

While it is often debated whether caffeine is good or bad for your health, there are numerous risks with drinking caffeine. Caffeine increases cortisol or "stress-hormone" levels; it disturbs sleep; it is dehydrating and can potentially create digestive issues. Caffeine is a natural stimulant found in coffees, teas, sodas and energy drinks. Many caffeinated beverages contain other pimple-promoting ingredients as well.

Consider this popular daily beverage scenario: large vanilla latte with cream, sugar and maybe a few pumps of vanilla.

Here's what you're really getting:

- The caffeine in the coffee increases the hormone cortisol. This disturbs your sleep and increases your androgen levels. It also dehydrates the body, increasing inflammation.

- The cream promotes inflammation and raises androgen levels increasing oil production. And if its not organic, it will disrupt your hormone and bacteria balance.
  - Substitute soymilk (thinking it's healthier) instead of cream. Soy is a hormone disrupter that increases insulin and causes inflammation.
  - Substitute cream for low-fat or fat-free dairy and create a sugar bomb. Taking the fat out of the dairy changes the ratio and creates a sugary drink causing spikes in the hormone insulin.

- Vanilla flavoring results in a sugar-feeding growth of bad bacteria, yeast, candida and increases insulin levels, all causing inflammation and potential hormonal imbalance.
  - Sugar-free sweeteners as a substitute for sugar are not a better alternative. Artificial sweeteners (including Stevia) alter the balance of your gut bacteria, increase inflammation, raise insulin levels and increase oil production.

Your daily coffee drink is a weapon of mass destruction and costs upwards of $5.00. Not only does the daily habit bust your budget, it can also bust your skin with acne.

My Recommendation: If you choose to consume caffeine, make sure it is organic and consumed early in the day. Black coffee is a best choice. If you have to have cream in it, remember to make sure to use organic whole milk. If you need a dairy substitute (rice, coconut, almond), make sure it does not have sweeteners, GMOs, carrageenan, artificial flavors and colors. No soy substituting.

HIGH-QUALITY H2O

The standard amount of water recommended is at least half your bodyweight in ounces of water per day (if you weigh 130 pounds, you should be drinking 65 ounces of water per day). If you work out, consume any alcohol or caffeinated beverages, or eat high amounts of protein, you will need to add additional amounts of water to cover the loss from sweat and dehydration. Seventy-five percent of Americans are chronically dehydrated. Even mild dehydration can put major stress on the body.

Dehydration causes the release of histamines. Histamines are a compound released in the body as a response to injury and allergic or inflammatory reactions. When the body is regularly releasing histamines, the result can be chronic inflammation. Histamines caused by dehydration can also cause false allergic reactions.

Dehydration also affects digestion. Your body needs water to produce stomach acid necessary for proper digestion. Low stomach acid can lead to protein malnourishment, mineral deficiencies, nutrient deficiencies, food sensitivities, leaky gut, an overgrowth of pathogens, and can create toxins. The negative effects of dehydration can trigger acne breakouts.

CLEARING CONFUSION ON WATER TYPES

Water is essential to life. There are different types, which can be confusing: spring, filtered, alkaline, tap and more. So, let's look at these:

- **Spring water** – This is the best type of water to drink, because it is naturally filtered by the earth and contains beneficial trace minerals. It should come from a protected source that is certified free from pollutants. (refer to "Additional Resources")

- **Distilled and filtered (purified) water** – This type of water, filtered and reverse osmosis, remove some of the harmful pollutants. However, they also strip the water of its minerals. Minerals help water absorb properly and are crucial to staying hydrated. Water is where we consume a large part of our daily mineral intake.

- **Alkaline water** – This type of water is ionized and less acidic. It contains alkalizing compounds like calcium, silica, potassium, magnesium and bicarbonate making it beneficial for hydration. On the other hand, it is possible to become too alkaline, which is harmful to the body. It will be necessary to regulate your consumption accordingly by measuring your pH. To determine your alkaline and acid levels you can use pH test strips.

- **Tap water** – This type of water, depending on where you live, may contain varying amounts of chlorine, fluorine, trihalomethanes (THMs), arsenic, aluminum, lead, mercury, nitrates, pesticides, drugs, and hormones to name a few. Some of these, like chlorine, are added in an attempt to make our drinking water "safe" for consumption. Chlorine, used to disinfect tap water, not only kills bad bacteria, but it also destroys intestinal flora. These friendly bacteria help to digest food, produce vitamins, absorb vitamins, reduce inflammation, and help with hormone production.

Chlorine internally and externally can lead to acne, eczema, rashes, sensitive skin and other skin irritations. It will also strip your hair and skin of its natural oils leading to dry, brittle hair and dry, flakey skin. Chlorine promotes free radicals in the body and skin. Free radicals and chlorine are cancer causing.

Tap water is linked to bladder, breast, and bowel cancer. Long-term effects of drinking, bathing and swimming in chlorinated water has been shown to cause malignant melanoma, aka SKIN CANCER! Free radicals within the skin promote the aging process just like sun exposure does, resulting in premature aging and fine lines. Unless you live in a place that is known for its healthy tap water, DO NOT drink it.

My Recommendation: As stated, spring water is the best choice for drinking water. I sometimes alternate between alkaline and spring water to ensure that I am staying hydrated. The best way to drink water is warm or at room temperature because it is more easily absorbed by your body than drinking cold water.

CHAPTER 5.
Nutritional Supplements for Acne

Dietary supplements can improve your health, but are not intended to replace eating nutritious foods rich in vitamins, minerals, antioxidants, enzymes, fiber and more. Consider supplements instead as an insurance policy on your health.

Most people do not get proper nutrition from what they eat in a typical day, and it is not always because of poor eating habits. The quality of our food has drastically declined over the past fifty years. Even healthful foods like fruits, vegetables and meats have been raised/grown in depleted soils, have added pesticides and hormones, have been genetically modified (GMO), have been over-processed, contain food additives, and are packaged with material containing environmental – toxins that are contributing to the rise of many serious health conditions, including acne.

KNOW YOUR SUPPLEMENTS

Many supplements are made out of synthetic materials and contain gluten and other additives, which cause a low absorption rate due to a lack of quality or poor gut health. This does not mean we shouldn't take supplements; it means you need to be more selective and aware of what you put into your body.

Being selective is choosing whole-food supplements that are non-GMO and free of gluten, dairy, soy, corn, sugar, artificial colors, sweeteners, titanium dioxide, stearic acid and cellulose powder. Be sure you check packaging is BPA-free, too.

While supplements like A, C, E, zinc, magnesium and selenium are considered star nutrients in curing acne, in truth, all vitamins either directly or indirectly aid in the reduction of acne. The following sections highlight specific types of supplements that help clear acne.

NOTE: Unless you have identified a specific deficiency, avoid taking large doses of any supplement. Some supplements can have harmful interactions with certain types of medications. Consult with your doctor if you have any health conditions, are pregnant, nursing, or are on any prescription medications before taking any supplements.

MULTIVITAMIN SUPPLEMENTS

Multivitamin and multi-mineral supplements help boost your nutrient intake and promote radiant, clear skin. Taking vitamins and minerals in combination with other specific nutrients promotes better absorption. For example, taking Vitamin D with Calcium increases absorption. It's important to find a multivitamin that is a good quality i.e. it's standardized, it's a whole-food supplement (not synthetic), and it's free from gluten and fillers.

My Recommendation: Multivitamins are better utilized in doses instead of the one-a-day formulas. To avoid feeling nauseous, make sure to take a multivitamin with food.

PROBIOTICS AND PREBIOTICS

There are thousands of different species of bacteria living in our bodies. Different strains of bacteria provide different health benefits. Probiotics are living bacteria and yeasts that are good for your general health and digestive system. Prebiotics are indigestible fiber that fuel good bacteria.

Soil-based organisms (SBOs) are a different class of probiotics that also help to balance and support our microbiomes. To repopulate the gut with good bacteria and reestablish a healthy lining or barrier, a wide variety of strains are best. Prebiotics and probiotics work together to reduce inflammation, lower stress, improve digestion, balance hormones and are essential for improving and clearing acne.

My Recommendation: Deciding which pre- and probiotics to buy can be overwhelming. When choosing a probiotic formula, look for labeling with a high CFU (colony-forming unit) count, such as 25-50 billion, and strain diversity of 15 or more, has prebiotics (food for probiotics), SBOs if possible, survivability (resists stomach acid), is shelf–stable and heat resistant. Buy organic if you can. I advise against getting probiotics from yogurt. Yogurt is a dairy product and usually contains sugar with minimal strains of good bacteria and not enough CFUs (refer to "Additional Resources").

OMEGA-3 FATTY ACID

Omega-3 fatty acids like Docosahexaenoic Acid (DHA) and Eicosapentaenoic Acid (EPA) help reduce inflammation, decrease insulin resistance, balance cortisol levels, decrease oil production and reduce the skin's susceptibility to sun damage, preventing pigmentation and premature wrinkling. The standard recommended dose is 1000 mg per day. Because many Western diets contain high Omega-6 fatty acids (pro-inflammatory) to Omega-3 fatty acids (anti-inflammatory) ratio, eating foods rich in Omega-3 fatty acids can help provide balance.

My Recommendation: Eat foods such as salmon, sardines, egg yolks, avocados, almonds, walnuts, flaxseed, and olive and coconut oils to help balance fatty acids.

VITAMIN D

The natural and optimal form of Vitamin D is D3, also known as cholecalciferol. Vitamin D is actually a hormone that is essential for strong bones and helps reduce inflammation, strengthens the immune system and normalizes sebum production. Vitamin D is produced by the body in response to exposure to sunlight. It can also be consumed by eating egg yolks, beef liver, certain fish and fish oils, and fortified milk products. People who are at higher risk of Vitamin D deficiency include people who follow a strict vegan diet, have little exposure to sunlight, have darker skin tones, kidney problems or digestive issues.

My Recommendation: Request a blood test from your doctor to assess your Vitamin D levels before supplementing beyond the maximum recommended daily limit of 5000 IU. To naturally get D3, eat salmon, sardines, egg yolks and dark leafy greens.

TURMERIC

Turmeric, also known as curcumin, is a member of the ginger family and has been used in traditional Chinese and Indian medicine for thousands of years. Taken internally, it can reduce inflammation and insulin sensitivity, which are major risk factors contributing to acne. Turmeric can also support gut health.

My Recommendation: Dr. Perlmutter, author of the book *Grain Brain,* advises supplementing with 500 mg twice a day. Make sure you find a supplement that is standardized, includes the full spectrum of curcuminoids and is enhanced with bioperine to ensure proper absorption.

CHAPTER 6.
Detox Your Body

Eliminating toxins is the first step in detoxing your body and healing your acne. Exposure to toxins is everywhere – in the air, water, soil, food and consumer products. Environmental toxins are both man-made and naturally occurring chemicals that are harmful to your health.

Toxins get into your home and into your body, often under the assumption products are safe. Toxins occur in non-organic foods, non-filtered water, microwaving, cleaning products, chlorine bleach, antibacterial soap, beauty products, paint, building supplies, chemicals, carpet, candles, dry cleaning and home air fresheners, to name a few.

We are slowly being poisoned and most of us are oblivious or think it's no big deal. Not only do we have to worry about outside toxins, even our own bodies excrete harmful endotoxins due to bad bacteria in our system that can disrupt healthy skin.

While some toxic products and byproducts create immediate reactions, others are seemingly harmless. But, ongoing exposure to these poisons over time creates a toxic burden on our bodies. Instead of the body eliminating toxins naturally, they can get stored in our fat cells and tissues in an attempt to protect our vital organs from damage. There comes a tipping point where an array of negative side effects triggers a domino effect that can manifest into serious health problems and skin problems like acne, rosacea and/or eczema.

ORGANS OF DETOXIFICATION

There are five main organs involved in the detoxification or elimination process, including the lungs, liver, kidneys, intestines and skin. If our bodies are to survive this environment, these organs must work together seamlessly.

The **liver** is the primary detoxification organ in the body and involved in over 200 other separate functions and processes. It breaks down, deactivates and removes food additives, chemical pollutants and toxic medications that we may have ingested. The liver cleanses the blood and discharges waste products, aids in the digestive process and maintains hormone balance. It also manufactures cells to filter and destroy foreign invaders like bacteria, fungi, viruses and cancerous cells.

Too much protein, simple carbohydrates, alcohol, heavy metals, pesticides and other toxins in our diets, as well as lack of exercise, cause inflammation and harm the liver. An unhealthy or leaky gut also harms the liver allowing endotoxins into the bloodstream. The overworked liver begins to create hormonal imbalances as a result of the toxic overload. One thing leads to the next and toxicity creeps into all areas of the body, causing damage little by little.

The **kidneys** are two bean-shaped organs that are essential for keeping our bodies in balance. Kidneys filter our blood of toxic waste and excess water, balance body fluids and sodium (essential for healthy blood pressure regulation and neurological system), form urine, and aid in other important functions of the body. They reside against the back muscles in the upper abdominal cavity.

The **lungs** (our respiratory system) supply oxygen to our blood and remove carbon dioxide and other toxins that are produced through normal chemical reactions in our body through breathing. Acetaldehyde, the chemical created when the liver destroys alcohol (the smell on the breath of someone who has consumed a lot of alcohol), is just one example of gas that would be lethal if not expelled through the lungs. Phlegm is another way our bodies try to eliminate toxins.

The **intestines** are a long, continuous tube running from the stomach to the anus that help to break down food, absorb nutrients and eliminate waste and toxins. When the large intestine, also referred to as the colon or large bowel, is unable to remove waste (feces) from your body efficiently, it creates an unhealthy bowel and can lead to autointoxication. Autointoxication is poisoning caused by toxins in fecal matter being absorbed by the colon wall and re-circulated through the blood stream. The lymphatic system, liver, lungs and kidneys can become overburdened putting your body at risk for serious health problems.

The **skin** is the largest organ in our body that protects us from the outside world. It is also an eliminatory organ with sweat glands to flush out toxins and excess minerals from the body. When any one the organs involved in detoxification aren't working properly, it can cause an excess build-up of toxins in the body showing up in the form of itching, acne, eczema or other skin rashes, including rosacea and psoriasis.

Symptoms that indicate you may need detoxification include fatigue, skin rashes, itching, acne (especially hormonal), eczema, digestion problems (bloating, constipation, diarrhea), bad breath, headaches, PMS, hormonal imbalance, irregular period cycles, infertility, brain fog, weight gain or inability to lose weight, chronic muscle or joint pain and inflammatory conditions/diseases.

DETOXIFICATION STRATEGIES

Detoxification can be accomplished safely and easily by eating nutrient-dense foods and reducing your exposure to toxins. Below is a list of additional detoxification strategies:

- Eat nutrient-dense foods.
- Reduce and eliminate exposure to toxins.
- Take specific supplements to aide in detoxification.
- Fast/juice.
- Reduce potential allergens/allergy-causing food groups.
- Reduce candida overgrowth in the body.
- Reduce or eliminate prescriptions and OTC medications.
- Replace household cleaning products, toiletries and cosmetics with non-toxic alternatives.
- Increase exercise.
- Start dry body brushing.
- Take Epsom salt baths.
- Begin colonics and coffee enemas.
- Use FAR infrared sauna therapy.

DETOXIFICATION SUPPLEMENTS

Silymarin, the primary active compound in milk thistle, is an herb that has been used for over 2,000 years to treat many different health concerns. Milk thistle is an antioxidant that reduces inflammation, promotes healthy digestive function, decreases blood sugar levels, improves insulin resistance and is most well known for being a natural liver detoxifier. It can help liver problems, including cirrhosis, and decrease damage to the liver caused by heavy metals, prescription medications, antibiotics, alcohol and so on.

Milk thistle helps guard against the depletion of glutathione, a master antioxidant that helps to protect the body from disease formation and slow the aging process. Milk thistle is great for the skin, helping to prevent skin cancer and visible signs of aging like dark spots (liver spots), hyperpigmentation and fine lines and wrinkles.

Recommendation: Find a supplement with 80% pure, milk-thistle extract. Take anywhere between 50 ml to 150 ml two to three times daily, depending on whether you are using it for maintenance or during a detox program. Milk thistle is generally safe, but can have some interactions with certain medications, including blood thinners or allergy medications.

Glutathione is a peptide present in every cell in the body. It is the body's most powerful and important antioxidant because it provides the greatest protection against disease and premature aging. Glutathione helps to detoxify our cells and the liver, removes heavy metals, toxins and free radicals, strengthens the immune system, improves energy, improves athletic performance and recovery, slows down the aging process and improves the skin.

Increasing glutathione levels will help improve skin by minimizing age spots, discoloration and wrinkles. Glutathione has a skin-whitening effect from the inside vs. topical whiteners (bleaching cream) that reduce uneven pigment after the fact.

Recommendation: Foods that contain glutathione are only uncooked cruciferous vegetables (broccoli, Brussel sprouts, cabbage, kale), fruit, unpasteurized dairy, raw eggs and raw meats. Once you cook, pasteurize or process these foods, little to no glutathione is left.

Unfortunately, glutathione supplements are not absorbed well by the body. If you decide to take it in supplemental form, make sure you choose Liposomal Glutathione (200 mg – 500 mg daily) or Acetylated Glutathione (200 mg – 500 mg daily S-Acetylated form). Otherwise, you can boost glutathione levels by taking certain supplements like N-Acetyl Cysteine (NAC), Alpha Lipoic Acid (ALA) and eating certain foods.

N-Acetyl Cysteine (NAC) – NAC is another antioxidant that helps rid the body of free radicals and peroxides. It is also a precursor to glutathione production and has broad health benefits. NAC improves insulin sensitivity, blocks cancer development, fights Helicobacter Pylori, reduces oxidative stress linked to inflammation, slows down the aging process, and improves cell health in the liver, skin, hair, and eyes. It slows down the aging process and improves your skin, hair, nails and eyes. It can help reduce the appearance of blemishes, age spots and wrinkles.

Recommendations: NAC is not found naturally in foods, therefore, it is an altered form of cysteine that the body converts to glutathione. Foods rich in cysteine are high protein foods. NAC is generally considered safe with some potential stomach-related side effects such as nausea, diarrhea or constipation.

There is no standard recommended dose established, so anywhere between 600 -1,800 mg per day seems to be effective. With this in mind, I recommend starting with a smaller dose with food two times per day and gradually increase to avoid any potential stomach upset.

Alpha Lipoic (ALA) is both water and fat-soluble making it a powerful and universal antioxidant. ALA also up-regulates glutathione levels by regenerating other antioxidants. It helps to improve adrenal output, improves insulin sensitivity, protects against Leaky Gut Syndrome, supports liver detoxification, reduces inflammation in the body and helps to reduce autoimmune activity. ALA is beneficial for skin because it helps to reduce inflammation (swelling, puffiness, redness, blotchiness) and creates more even skin tone.

Recommendations: Foods that contain ALA are cruciferous vegetables, organ meats (beef or chicken liver, hearts, kidneys), tomatoes, peas, beets and carrots. There are no established doses; however, 300 – 600 ml per day on an empty stomach is recommended for healthy adults. Make sure you look for the R-ALA form and avoid the S-ALA form or a combination of both.

Larger doses can be taken to help with specific health concerns, but it needs to be determined and monitored by the treating doctor. ALA may be contraindicated for certain medications (to lower blood sugar, antibiotics, anti-inflammatories). Side effects include nausea and skin rashes, but are rare and mild.

Selenium is a trace mineral that acts like an antioxidant helping to neutralize free radicals. It helps prevent coronary heart disease, helps maintain thyroid related hormones, detoxifies the body, strengthens the immune system, reduces inflammation, boosts hair growth and helps heal acne. Selenium protects the skin's elasticity and protects it from the sun by neutralizing free radicals and other skin damaging compounds before they can lead to wrinkles. It also helps to prevent the inflammation of acne, eczema and psoriasis.

Recommendations: Foods that contain selenium include Brazil nuts, sunflower seeds, chia seeds, eggs, liver, rockfish, tuna, herring, chicken breast, salmon, turkey and mushrooms. Avoid taking high levels of selenium, as it can lead to selenium poisoning and potentially be fatal. Selenium deficiency is rare in the United States so unless you are under the care of a physician recommending higher doses, the standard supplement dose is 55 micrograms daily. Eating a diet rich in the foods listed above will prevent the need to take any additional supplementation.

MSM (methylsulfonylmethane) is a sulfur-based compound and an essential nutrient found in an array of natural unprocessed foods. MSM is a crucial beauty nutrient. It helps with collagen and keratin production necessary to heal the skin and acne scarring. MSM helps produce skin flexibility, detoxifies the body, heals gastrointestinal problems, increases absorption of nutrients, and is anti-inflammatory.

My Recommendation: Foods rich in sulfur are arugula, broccoli, Brussels sprouts, cabbage, cauliflower, kale, radish, turnip, watercress, eggs and sea vegetables. If you choose to supplement with MSM, it will be better absorbed in powder form and in conjunction with antioxidants like Vitamin C. Make sure the MSM formula does not contain synthetic byproducts and fillers.

Start with one to two tablespoons of the powder or crystal form of MSM mixed with water and gradually increase dosage as your body gets used to it to avoid digestive side effects. Unfortunately, it tastes quite bitter. I mix mine in a small glass of juice and drink it quickly to mask any unpleasant taste. Ideally, this should be taken on an empty stomach. Side effects of MSM supplements include nausea, diarrhea and abdominal discomfort.

Chlorella's protein levels and combination of vitamins, minerals, phytonutrients and phytochemicals make it one of the most nutrient-dense, super foods in the world. It detoxifies heavy metals, supports your immune system, promotes weight loss, fights cancer, lowers blood sugar and cholesterol, and protects your skin from premature aging by increasing levels of Vitamin A, Vitamin C and glutathione in your body.

Recommendations: Chlorella can come in pill or powder form. Adding chlorella powder to smoothies is a great way to supplement your diet. Make sure to purchase a formula that contains "cracked cell-wall chlorella" so your body is able to absorb it easily. Common chlorella side effects include diarrhea, nausea, green stools, and stomach cramping, especially in the first week of use.

However, these side effects are typical of any detoxification program. I would start slow and gradually increase the amount of chlorella to allow your body to adjust and minimize potential side effects. People can have serious allergic reactions to taking chlorella, especially if they are allergic to iodine.

Activated charcoal, also called activated carbon, is a form of carbon processed to have small, low-volume pores that increase the surface area available for absorption or chemical reactions. This is not to be confused with the charcoal in your barbecue grill. Used to treat poisoning and drug overdose, activated charcoal prevents the absorption of certain drugs by binding to toxins to help rid the body of unwanted substances. Activated charcoal can alleviate gas and bloating, filter and clean water, help the body flush out toxins, support digestive cleansing, whiten teeth and improve skin's health.

Recommendations: Purchase activated charcoal made from coconut shells. If you choose the powdered form, make sure there are no artificial sweeteners. Activated charcoal can cause dehydration, so be sure to drink plenty of water with it to avoid constipation and help flush out toxins quickly. It can also bind to and interfere with the absorption of nutrients, supplements and prescription medications, so be sure to take it at least two hours prior to any of these. Activated charcoal can also have adverse interactions with certain drugs, so be sure to look them up before you start supplementing.

A BREAK FROM COOKING – FASTING

Fasting usually refers to abstaining from some or all kinds of food or drink for a specified period of time. There are a multitude of fasting programs including water, juicing and bone-broth versions that offer both healing and prevention, since the body expends significant energy on digestion.

Fasting has been used in health recovery for thousands of years. When you fast, your body undergoes physiological rest that allows it to focus on detoxification. Fasting aids in healing your gut, balancing your insulin levels, and reducing inflammation.

However, the theory behind fasting is controversial. Some experts believe it is harmful to your health. For example, certain medical conditions, such as pregnancy and hypoglycemia, are not conducive to fasting. Fasting is also not recommended when on certain medications.

My Recommendation: It's always a good idea to consult with your doctor on any health issues or medication before beginning any type of fasting regimen.

TIMING AND DURATION

The type and length of fast you choose depends on your goals, health, and circumstances. A one-day or a 24-hour fast is a good way to begin if you have never fasted before. It can be as simple as stop eating after 6 p.m. on Tuesday and resume eating after 6 p.m. on Wednesday. Three-day fasts are ideal over weekends, especially because they keep the weekend free for bed rest if needed. Three-day fasts help eliminate toxins and clear your blood. One-week fasts or 10-day fasts are reserved for quarterly (seasonal) practice and not only eliminate toxins and clean your blood, but begin healing and rebuilding your body.

INTERMITTENT FASTING

Intermittent fasting is gaining in popularity as a safe method of fasting that is shorter and easier to do on a regular basis. This type of fasting splits the day or week into eating and fasting periods. Intermittent fasting is consuming your calories during a smaller specific window of the day. Intermittent fasting promotes weight loss and muscle building, helps to balance insulin levels, and allows the body to use fat stored in the body as energy.

You can adjust this fasting window depending on work hours, when you exercise and family meals. Because it is so flexible, you can customize it to work for your life. Some example fasting protocols:

- If you start eating at 8 a.m., stop eating at 4 p.m.
- If you start eating at 11 a.m., stop eating at 7 p.m.

You can also shorten the period of time you are allowed to eat called feasting. Example:

- If you start eating at 2 p.m., stop eating at 8 p.m.

Some people practice intermittent fasting daily. If not done correctly, intermittent fasting can cause hormonal imbalance in women. Women are extremely sensitive to signals of starvation. Hunger hormones leptin and ghrelin will increase in the body when these hormones sense that it's being starved. For beginners, and for women, start with crescendo fasting. This type of fasting is done 2 to 3 non-consecutive days per week. For example, you can fast intermittently on Tuesday, Thursday and maybe Saturday. Once your body has adjusted to this method (in 2 to 4 weeks), you can add an additional day if you want to.

My Recommendation: This is the type of fasting I practice on a regular basis. It is the easiest and least invasive to the body, so this is where I would start if I wanted to attempt fasting.

JUICE FASTING

Juicing and juice fasting have become very popular over the past few decades. Fruits and vegetables are anti-inflammatory and loaded with antibacterial nutrients to help heal the body as well as repair the skin.

My Recommendation: Avoid juicing with fruit as it is nothing more than a sugar bomb. Green vegetables are the lowest in sugar and should make up the bulk of your juice. Also, consuming protein during juice fasting is ideal because it aides in the detoxification process.

Great sources of protein include spirulina, hemp seeds, ground flax seeds, chia seeds or a vegan protein powder that is free of sugar, wheat, gluten, corn, dairy and peanuts. Certain vegetables and fruits contain some protein.

Some examples are avocados, kale, spinach, Brussels sprouts, broccoli, cantaloupe, strawberries, watermelon and oranges. Adding herbs like turmeric, ginger and/or cilantro will enhance your detoxification process. Be sure to buy organic, so you are not ingesting pesticides and other toxic chemicals.

BONE-BROTH FASTING

Bone broth is nothing new. It has been around as long as humans have had fire. Our ancestors knew what they were doing when they made chicken soup for colds and flus. Bone broth is made with beef, turkey, chicken or fish bones and water. Simmering these bones releases healing compounds of amino acids, collagen and trace minerals that help repair your gut and are beneficial for your skin's appearance. It is typically simmered anywhere from four to 24 hours, depending upon the type of bones you use.

My Recommendation: Purchase grass-fed beef, pasture-raised chicken and/or wild-caught fish, not farmed. Bouillon cubes (artificial-flavor salt blocks) along with canned and boxed broth, are not acceptable substitutes for making bone broth. You can purchase genuine bone broth online, but it is very expensive. Making it at home is much more cost effective, and in my opinion, tastes much better (refer to "Additional Resources").

WATER FASTING

Water fasting is just what it sounds like, water only. Water fasting allows your digestive system to rest completely. People detox, heal and burn fat quickly with water fasting. While water fasting is the most challenging, it produces the quickest and most therapeutic results. If you have any health concerns or intend to water fast for more than three days, it should be done under the supervision of a health-care professional.

If fasting is not your thing, just eating an organic anti-inflammatory diet, reducing your exposure to environmental toxins in your home, and using non-toxic personal-care products is really a whole-body cleanse in and of itself.

ALLEVIATE ALLERGIES

An allergy is an immune response by the body to an irritant (food, pollen, fur, mold, parasites, etc.). Allergies can be mild to severe. They can have an immediate response or be delayed and can be seasonal or year-round. Symptoms can range from hives, to itchy eyes or nose, to sneezing. Some symptoms, seemingly unrelated, can show up in the form of acne, eczema, fatigue, weight gain, headaches, nausea and dark circles under the eyes to name a few. It is quite possible your acne is related to an allergy of which you are unaware.

So, how do you know if you have an allergy if it is not immediate and obvious? Request a food allergy or food sensitivity test from your doctor. There are a few different types of food- allergy tests to choose from. The two most popular are skin-prick testing and blood testing. For acne, I would recommend a blood test that measures both IgG and IgE. The two together are more comprehensive than either one alone. Which allergy test the doctor chooses depends on each person's unique circumstances such as symptoms, severity of allergy, cost, and time. These tests are not always 100% accurate, but I would still recommend doing one. It is possible to test negative for a food sensitivity/allergy that you actually do have.

These tests can yield helpful information regarding which foods and other irritants are causing inflammation, so you can cut down or completely stop your exposure to them. It is my guess that if your test results come back with moderate sensitivities to many foods and irritants, you may have leaky gut. Repair the gut and get rid of some, if not all, of your food allergies. This will help to reduce your acne.

If you are unable to obtain food-allergy testing or tests are inconclusive, try doing the Whole30™ diet. This diet eliminates the most common food allergens helping you reduce your exposure to potential allergens and allow your gut to begin healing.

KILL CANDIDA

Candida albicans is a species of yeast (aka fungus) that lives in various parts of the body, including the digestive tract. It can coexist peacefully with other bacteria and yeast, but if a small population gets out of control, it can affect your health. Toxic metabolites produced by candida lead to gut inflammation and gut inflammation can increase the growth of candida.

Candida can cause skin problems by causing or contributing to leaky gut, which, as I already covered, has a link to skin health. People with acne and other skin conditions have been found to have higher levels of candida antibodies in their blood, suggesting leaky gut as well. Overgrowth of candida can cause the immune system to overreact inducing an inflammatory response, triggering the acne-formation process.

What can you do to decrease your candida and balance your intestinal flora? Use a nutrition plan that is low sugar, gluten-free, and anti-inflammatory (for starters). A diet high in vegetable fiber will feed healthy bacteria and encourage production of a substance that reduces inflammation called butyrate.

NOTE: Antifungal medications may be necessary in some cases. However, if the way you eat doesn't change, candida will eventually return along with your acne. If you want additional assistance in cleansing your body, there are cleansing supplements that will provide specific nutrients to help to kill candida, support the liver in detoxification, bind toxins and gently remove the captured toxins through the digestive tract and out of the body.

GET OFF THE DRUGS

While some medications can be lifesaving, just because a doctor prescribed a treatment doesn't mean you need to blindly accept everything he or she says . Be aware of what you put into your body and make choices about what is best for you after weighing pros and cons. For example: many prescription medications, over-the-counter medications and some dietary supplements contain fillers like gluten, wheat, corn, soy and toxic chemicals that can cause skin problems, among many other negative side effects.

Some medications have an acne-promoting side effect. Medications to be aware of include anabolic steroids (testosterone), corticosteroids (Prednisone), lithium and bromides (inhalers and nasal sprays). Supplements like DHEA and excess B vitamins (B1, B6 and B12) can promote acne flare-ups as well. Anti-inflammatory pain medicines like aspirin, ibuprofen, and naproxen are hard on the liver and all damage the intestinal lining, which leads to inflammation and can result in acne.

NOTE: I am not suggesting you stop taking prescribed and necessary medications. However, dietary modifications and/or natural remedies can often be implemented as an alternative to dangerous prescription drugs and OTCs.

Do not expect your traditional allopathic doctors to suggest these other remedies because they are not educated in natural medicine. Allopathic refers to our mainstream medical system that aims to combat disease by use of drugs or surgery as opposed to naturopathic medicine that emphasizes prevention, treatment and optimal health through the use of therapeutic methods and substances that encourage the individuals' inherent self-healing process.

What's worse, they may even poo-poo the idea of natural remedies such as diet and lifestyle changes in lieu of medication. Not to mention the drug companies don't "push" natural remedies and supplements because they don't make any money from the sale of those!

In truth, it does seem easier to take medication rather than changing your eating habits and exercising. But the result is usually sub-par to nutritional changes. What's worse is medications can mask the problem, while the root cause is allowed to continue to cause further damage to your system, resulting in more health problems.

My Recommendation: Unless it is a matter of life or death, try modifying your diet and lifestyle first. Investigate all prescriptions and their potential side effects before you just start taking them. An estimated 128,000 Americans die every year as a result of taking prescribed medications, excluding overdose and misuse. OTC medications are potentially harmful as well.

Do not assume because a prescription is not required that it is safe for short-term or long-term use. My advice is to get a naturopathic doctor in addition to the doctor your insurance covers. Only then you can make an informed choice as to which medications are necessary.

GET OFF YOUR BUTT

Exercise is great for your body and your skin. Light to moderate exercise and physical activity increases blood flow to your dermis (skin), opens up the pores, releases oils and toxins, and help to decrease stress hormone levels that influence oil production and inflammation that cause acne. Circulation helps nourish and heal acne by delivering oxygen and nutrients to skin cells and carrying away waste. Exercise, if not excessive, lowers blood sugar levels, normalizes insulin levels, increases the production and release of serotonin, dopamine, cortisol, testosterone and growth hormone, which all aid to healthy skin. Exercise leads to lipolysis, helping release toxins that are stored in our fat cells.

Bear in mind that exercise can put stress on the body. Excessive exercising, especially marathon running and/or intensive weight-lifting routines with little recovery time, can adversely affect cortisol, adrenaline levels and many other hormones. When hormones are regularly overproduced, blood sugar imbalances and chronic inflammation occur, which we already know contributes to acne. I am not telling you not to exercise. Exercise is good for acne, just do not overdo it.

Recommendations: Daily exercise is recommended for all ages. Anything from walking, to weight lifting, to house cleaning, to chasing small children, all counts as exercise. When exercising, wear loose-fitting clothing made from moisture-wicking fabrics or cotton to avoid causing chafing or friction from tight clothing and increased sweating that can cause acne. Avoid polyester and man-made fabrics that trap oil, sweat and bacteria. Do not wear makeup while working out. Wearing makeup while sweating increases the risk of clogged pores, trapping toxins, and stirring up inflammation. Showering immediately after can aid in preventing acne.

SWEAT IT OUT

FAR Infrared-sauna therapy uses infrared light waves that penetrate the skin and create heat in the body verses heating the air outside the body like traditional dry or steam saunas. FAR Infrared saunas are safe and usually tolerated much better than standard saunas. They help release stored toxins in the body, improve blood circulation, boost metabolism, decrease inflammation, increase wound healing and much more.

Recommendations: FAR Infrared saunas are safe to use every day and you will improve faster if you use it 30-45 minutes daily. (refer to "Additional Resources").

SCRUB IT OFF

Dry body brushing is an easy-to-do natural skin-care routine that exfoliates dead skin, unclogs pores, stimulates blood circulation, increases lymphatic drainage, reduces cellulite and excretes toxins that become trapped in the skin. Dry body brushing is performed dry with a natural bristle brush (not synthetic) with a long handle for hard-to-reach areas of the body.

Recommendations: Only dry brush your body a few times per week to avoid over-scrubbing and irritating the skin. Brush each area several times allowing for some overlap. Brush strokes should always go in the direction towards your heart.

TAKE AN EPSOM SALT BATH

Different from table salt, Epsom salt is a mineral compound of magnesium and sulfate. It has multiple uses and benefits for health and beauty. For starters, Epsom salt baths have stress-reducing benefits. Just taking a bath is relaxing all by itself. Add Epsom salt to your bath and it will help boost magnesium levels that are involved in many important roles in the body, including elimination of harmful toxins. The magnesium and sulfate work like reverse osmosis, pulling dangerous toxins out of the body.

Epsom salts also relieve constipation by working as a laxative to cleanse the colon of waste. Epsom salt baths can help to reduce pain and inflammation (the root of most diseases – especially the skin), and helps to heal cuts and bruises. The magnesium and sulfate help to improve blood sugar by assisting the body in producing and utilizing insulin. All of these benefits help relieve the body of stress as well.

Recommendations: Take as many Epsom salt baths as you can find time for.

GRAB SOME COFFEE

Coffee enemas were first made famous by the Gerson Institute in the 1950's. This is a key component of treating cancer patients, according to their protocol. Coffee enemas infuse coffee via the anus to help remove toxins accumulated in the liver and to remove free radicals from the bloodstream. Caffeine helps cleanse the liver by opening up blood vessels and increasing circulation and immunity. It opens up bile ducts and increases bile production helping to relieve digestive issues and improve gut health.

Recommendations: Coffee enemas are inexpensive and can be done in the comfort of your own home. All you need is an enema kit, fresh organic coffee (never decaf) and some peace and privacy. To find out more information on how to perform a coffee enema go to www.gersoninstitute.com. Coffee enemas are considered safe, provided you are not overdoing them or causing dehydration. If you are pregnant, nursing, or under a doctor's care for any health issue, check with your doctor first.

CALL THE PLUMBER

Colon cleansing, also known as colon therapy, colon hydrotherapy, or colonic irrigation is an alternative medical therapy that removes toxins from the colon and intestinal tract by removing accumulations of old feces out of the colon by sending gallons of water into the body through a tube inserted into a person's rectum. This process sounds horrible, but is actually painless (except for your pride) and can make a significant difference in helping your body rid itself of toxins.

Organic coffee can be added to the colonic to produce some of the same benefits as a coffee enema, but is not to be confused with a coffee enema. Probiotics can be added to your colonic to repopulate good bacteria.

Recommendations: Unless otherwise prescribed, a series of three colonics a couple times of year would be beneficial in supporting and maintaining body detoxification. Colonics are safe, assuming they are performed by a licensed, qualified person and are not done too frequently. The regulations for what constitutes a qualified person are different from state to state.

Colonic irrigation done too often can disrupt the bowel's normal flora and result in electrolyte depletion. Individuals with a history of diverticulitis, Crohn's disease, ulcerative colitis, colon surgery, severe hemorrhoids, kidney or heart disease should check with their doctors before considering colon hydrotherapy.

CHAPTER 7.
Detox Your Home

In the earlier section on detoxifying your body, I mentioned the many ways toxins creep into our modern lives and compromise our health. If your home is like the average household, you can probably open your kitchen and bathroom cabinets and find dozens of chemicals that contribute to a poisonous environment. It is difficult for our bodies to eliminate these toxins naturally; instead, they are stored in our tissues and fat cells and eventually cause health problems, including acne, rosacea and eczema.

Cleaning products are not meant to be ingested, so they are not regulated by the Food and Drug Administration. The Environmental Working Group (EWG) reports that there are no safety standards regarding the ingredients in cleaning products. Manufacturers are only required by law to carry a list of "chemicals of known concern" on their labels. The FDA does not test, nor do they require the manufacturers to test these chemicals. The fact is that many "unknown" chemicals and "chemicals of known concern" used short and long term are harmful. Do not assume that products of any kind that you purchase are safe for you and your family to be using.

Similarly, the FDA does not regulate cosmetic products and their ingredients with the exception of color additives. Even if the product itself is "safe," it is possible the method of manufacturing/production is not. Accurate labeling and identification of potential harmful interactions with other variables are all things to consider in deciding if a product is safe. The beauty industry is for the most part unregulated and there are no legal standards for cosmetics labeled "organic," "pure," or "natural." You will need to do your own research and read labels carefully.

My Recommendation: When in doubt about a product, consult the EWG. By definition, The Environmental Working Group (EWG) is an American environmental organization that specializes in research and advocacy in the areas of toxic chemicals, agricultural subsidies, public lands, and corporate accountability. There is also a downloadable application called *Think Dirty* that rates a cosmetic and personal hygiene product's safety and offers cleaner alternatives where available. It may not have every product you're trying to look up, but they do a darn good job of helping consumers weed out the most harmful personal care items.

THE UNCLEAN 19

Some of the more common environmental toxins in products we use on our bodies and in our homes include the following:

1. **Bisphenol (BPA)** is in plastics such as water bottles and food packaging. To avoid it, use glass whenever possible.

2. **Oxybenzone** is a chemical used in sunscreens and cosmetics to block the sun's rays. Use physical sun blocks that contain minerals like zinc and titanium.

3. **Fluoride** is in tap water and toothpaste. For drinking water, use spring, alkaline or purified water and look for non-fluoride toothpastes.

4. **Parabens** are synthetic preservatives found in skin-care products, cosmetics, shampoos and conditioners. Look for paraben-free products.

5. **Phthalates** are used in plastics and are found in detergents, toys, cosmetics, food packaging, flooring, household fragrances, toilet paper, pharmaceuticals, deodorants and more. Look for phthalate-free products.

6. **Butylated hydroxyanisole (BHA) and its chemical counterpart, Butoxyethanol (BHT)** are preservatives found in processed foods, butter, meats, sausage, poultry, chewing gum, vegetable oils and beer, not to be confused with beta hydroxy acids used for facial peels. Avoid them.

7. **Perfluorooctanoic Acid (PFOA)** is in Teflon and non-stick coatings (pots and pans). It is also found in tap water. Use cooking utensils that don't have non-stick coatings.

8. **Perchlorate** is an oxidant found in drinking water and soil used to grow some of our vegetables. Buy organic produce and use spring, alkaline or purified water.

9. **Perchlorethylene** is found in dry-cleaning solutions, carpet and upholstery cleaners, shoe polish, adhesives, and wood cleaners. Check for EPA approvals on products.

10. **Triclosan** is found in soaps labeled "antibacterial". Avoid it.

11. **Quaternary Ammonium compounds "QUATS"** are found in fabric softeners, and liquid and dryer sheets. Check labels and avoid.

12. **Chlorine** is found in cleaning products, whiteners, and water. Limit exposure as much as possible. Get a filter for your shower head, drink purified water, and buy non-chlorine whiteners.

13. **Formaldehyde** is found in nail polish, eyelash glues, soaps, hair gels, makeup, shampoos and deodorants. Look for formaldehyde-free products.

14. **Petroleum by-products** are in mineral oil, petrolatum, liquid paraffin, skin-care products and cosmetics, vitamins, detergents, fertilizers, candles, plastics, bandages, asphalt, fuel and synthetic material. Look for petroleum-free products.

15. **Lead** is in lipstick, toothpaste, paint, vinyl and plastic such as bibs, backpacks, car seats, lunch boxes, batteries, and hair dye. Look for lead-free products.

16. **Mercury** is in pharmaceuticals and pesticides, mascara, and some fish. Avoid pharmaceuticals as much as possible, eat organic and use "natural" home pesticides, and mercury-free mascara. Eat fish usually considered safe, such as catfish, flounder, haddock, herring, salmon, trout, whitefish and sardines.

17. **Acrylates** are contained in artificial nail products. Avoid them.

18. **Bromides (BVOs)** are found in inhalers and nasal sprays, and canned or bottled citrus drinks. Bromides are also in chemical compounds used in hot tubs, germicidal agents, pesticides, baked goods, flour, drinking water, plastics and personal-care products. Avoid contact with these products as much as possible.

19. **Decabromodiphenyl Ether (DECA)** is a flame retardant found in electronics, furniture and carpet, essentially everywhere in your home. You might be most familiar with asbestos. Avoid it and have it removed if found in your home.

NOTE: Just because a product says it is free from any of these toxic items doesn't mean the product is completely safe either.

I have not listed every environmental toxin or guaranteed that every suggestion I make is organic and perfectly healthy in every way. I do not claim to be an expert on environmental toxins, cosmetics or household ingredients. This detox checklist is meant to bring awareness to hidden toxins in your environment so you can make informed decisions.

Mind you, I do not live entirely toxin-free, because it is difficult, nor do I consider myself a hypocrite because I don't. The point here is that the older I get, the more I become aware and the better my choices are for my own and my family's health. I try to limit my exposure to toxins for what I consider absolute musts, but I am not perfect. In my own household:

- I use organic hair dye because I'm 100-percent gray, but just because it is organic hair dye doesn't make it totally healthy either.
- I try to limit my use of products with parabens, but I use a few beauty products that have them.
- I try to avoid BPAs, but still I occasionally drink out of plastic "BPA blah-blah-blah free" bottles, which I'm sure we'll discover later are toxic as well.
- I try to eat healthy, but occasionally have my all-time favorite meal that includes chips, salsa and a margarita at my favorite Mexican restaurant.

An easy way to begin detoxing your home is to start buying organic foods, natural cleaning products and cosmetics (refer to "Additional Resources"). The good news is that a good portion of these toxic substances can be easily avoided by simply changing what we buy for use personally and in our homes!

CHAPTER 8.
Stress Less and Beauty Rest

Physical, emotional and mental stress directly and indirectly affect acne. Relationships, family, money, finances, health, poor sleep, work and other responsibilities, poor nutrition, and/or how we look and feel all affect our levels of stress.

Stress produces cortisol, which is our main stress hormone. Chronic stress creates blood-sugar imbalances, reduces digestive and detoxification capabilities, increases inflammation and androgen levels, which all contribute to acne.

Stress can affect many hormones negatively and can trigger androgen production, which in turn increases the amount of oil skin secretes. More oil means a greater likelihood of acne flare ups. It's a vicious cycle.

Also, stress affects the digestive system by shutting down blood flow to our gut, decreases secretions needed to break down nutrients, increases acid in the stomach and causes inflammation of the gastrointestinal system. This leaves us more susceptible to infection because it blocks absorption of vital nutrients and can lead to leaky gut. Some stress is unavoidable, but chronic stress contributes to many serious health problems and aging just as fast as eating cheeseburgers and drinking beer every day.

STRESS-REDUCTION STRATEGIES

I have created a list of suggestions for reducing stress levels. Start first with whichever ones will be the easiest. If you are following an anti-inflammatory nutrition plan, you are already reducing all forms of stress, so you can check that one off the list and move your focus to the next item on the list:

- Follow an anti-inflammatory diet.

- Take suggested supplements.

- Detox your body and your home.

- Get quality sleep. Sleep allows your body to repair itself and normalize cortisol levels (more on this in the next section).

- Get plenty of exercise. Physical exercise produces endorphins that naturally elevate mood and reduces cortisol.

- Get regular massages. Massage produces endorphins, relaxes muscle tension, and increases circulation. If this is cost prohibitive, enlist a good friend or partner to trade massages.

- Breathe deeply and learn to meditate. You may not realize it, but it's likely you are not breathing properly; shallow breathing is a habit. Deep breathing and meditation (which requires deep breathing) reduces sleep problems, gastrointestinal problems, stress and anxiety. Take time to focus on your breath and learn to meditate.

- Maintain positive social connections and spend time with friends and loved ones for cultivating good endorphins. By the same token, step away from negativity, gossip, and people who drain your energy. The effects of cortisol are dramatic and long-lasting in the body. Positive comments and connections spur oxytocin, a feel-good hormone that elevates trust, collaboration, communication and reduces stress levels.

- Engage in human touch. Similar to getting massages, the value of human touch cannot be overstated. Physical contact and affection elevates oxytocin, "The Love Hormone," triggers the increase of serotonin, the happy hormone.

- Engage in a spiritual practice of your choice, which helps the immune system, regulates negative emotions and reduces stress. Spiritual practice does not have to be some form of organized religion. It can be as simple as regularly playing music, meditating, dancing, gardening, golfing, hiking or painting. Spiritual practice helps to keep you in the moment or the now – not stuck in your past or in fear of the future.

- Seek professional coaching, counseling or a mentor, whether it is a professional fitness trainer, life coach, business coach or therapeutic counselor to help control and deal with negative emotions or stressful life events.

- Do more of what you love and less of what you don't love. Take time to be creative and have fun.

- Express gratitude by shifting your focus away from what you perceive as wrong or not working in life. Keep in mind that what you focus your attention on expands. Choose wisely.

- Practice effective time management. Create and schedule blocks of time to complete specific tasks. For example, designate certain times of day to return all calls and emails, and banish technology interruptions in between. Leverage your time by delegating and paying for assistance when it makes sense. Simplifying your life creates more time and less need to multi-task.

- Declutter your living and work space. The more space you have the more you have to manage, which becomes a time vampire and creates stress. Less is more. Donate, sell, toss, and shred anything you do not love, never use, or don't need. Organize what you have left.

BEAUTY REST

Sleep is critical for healthy skin. It is essential for the regulation of normal biological processes. A good night's rest affects various hormonal mechanisms that have the potential to cause acne. Sleep deprivation releases excess cortisol, which not only creates a blood sugar imbalance and GI detoxification issues, but also breaks down skin collagen. It decreases production of Human Growth Hormone (HGH) that serves to keep skin thick and healthy.

Lack of sleep also tends to make you irritable, less alert and can attribute to weight gain, which can cause more stress. Studies report psychological stress is increased 14% for every hour of lost sleep.

BEAUTY REST STRATEGIES

I have created a list of suggestions for getting better rest. If you do nothing else, commit to a consistent bedtime. Studies have shown that the most restorative sleep happens between the hours of 10pm and 2am, and it is recommended that adults aged 26 – 64 years old should typically get 7 to 9 hours of sleep each night (refer to "Additional Resources"). The following additional suggestions are provided to help improve sleep:

- Keep your room cool. A cooler body temperature makes it easier to sleep.

- Maintain a sleep schedule. Try to go to bed and wake up at the same time every day.

- Keep the room dark. Night lights, outside lights, alarms and electronic lights all interfere with restful sleep.

- Sleep in a comfortable bed. A good mattress, pillows and sheets keep your body comfortable. One-third of your life is spent sleeping, so invest in a quality bed.

- Avoid heavy meals. Eating large meals before bed fires up your metabolism, makes it more difficult to sleep and can aggravate acid reflux (if you are prone to it).

- Keep an electronic curfew. Decide on a time when you will stop and put away phones, laptops and turn off the television.

- Create a bedtime ritual before going to sleep every night Indulge in a hot shower or bath, drink warm tea, read something uplifting, or make love.

- Avoid serious conversations. Do not have stressful or serious conversations before bed. When people are tired they have less ability to listen, problem solve creatively, or exercise good understanding.

- Journal your thoughts to help calm your mind before bedtime.

- Take natural sleep-aid supplements when necessary. Deficiencies in 5 HTP, melatonin and GABA can lead to sleep disruption, digestive disorders, excessive stress and depression. You can buy these supplements separately or all in one supplement. Ask your doctor or naturopath for recommendations.

CHAPTER 9.
Balance Your Hormones

Do imbalances in hormones really cause acne? The answer is yes. Imbalances in androgen levels, insulin levels, cortisol levels and thyroid levels can lead to acne.

But the real question is what causes hormone imbalances? The root cause of most hormone imbalances is lifestyle, diet, environmental toxins, medications, and leaky gut. In most cases, changing the way you eat and making some lifestyle changes can normalize hormone levels.

How do you know if your hormone levels are out of balance and how do you correct them? You can request specific hormone testing (blood, saliva or urine) from your doctor to determine if your hormone levels are within the standardized range. However, it is important to remember that the standardized range is just an average that may not be "your normal."

For example, having a hormone test that falls in the low or high end of the normal range may actually be abnormal for you. It is also important, if you decide to get your hormones tested, to get a comprehensive hormone panel. Test for all three estrogens, progesterone, testosterone, in addition to DHA, DHEA, SHBG, cortisol, thyroid and insulin to provide a comprehensive report of hormone levels and their ratio to one another. For all you men, yes, you have estrogen and progesterone too! For females, it is also important to test at the proper time in your menstrual cycle and possibly time of day for each hormone you're testing.

There are many ways to balance your hormones should you find out you have an imbalance. The simplest way, with fewest side effects, least risk and more permanent, lasting results are dietary and lifestyle modifications. Make these changes and the problem usually resolves itself. Even if the hormone balance does not totally resolve itself, it will be less imbalanced and require less supplementation or medications, which will always be better for the body.

Bio-identical hormone replacement (HRT) can be very helpful in creating balance. However, changing your diet and lifestyle helps to balance hormones too. At the very least, diet and lifestyle modification may lessen the dose or frequency of HRT. Never attempt to balance your hormones with medications or supplements without proper testing first (more on HRT later).

INSULIN

Insulin is a hormone produced by the pancreas that helps regulate glucose in the blood and is essential for the metabolism of carbohydrates. All carbohydrates eventually get converted to glucose, and insulin turns glucose into fuel or body fat. If you eat more carbohydrates than your body needs, over time this causes your cells to become less sensitive and insulin resistant, causing high blood-sugar levels and inflammation.

To cope with high sugar, your body pumps out too much insulin to store as much glucose as possible. The stress hormone cortisol also increases insulin levels. Too much insulin can directly and indirectly cause acne. Insulin stimulates the production of sebum and increases the sensitivity of your skin's androgen receptors, increasing break-outs. It also enhances the ability of DHT to increase sebum production. Basically there is not a hormone in the body that is not affected or controlled by insulin. It is behind almost all hormonal imbalances.

There are many symptoms of insulin imbalance, including elevated blood sugar, abdominal obesity, fatty liver, increased risk of gout and kidney stones, high blood pressure, fluid retention (that gives you that puffy look), scalp hair loss on the front and sides in women, polycystic ovarian syndrome, large pores and acne.

It's a good idea to have your insulin levels (A1C test) and blood sugar levels (Fasting Blood Glucose Test) checked if you have persistent acne. The Fasting Blood Glucose Test measures current blood sugar levels. The A1C Test measures average blood sugar over the past two to three months, which provides a better picture of what's really going on.

Metformin is a popular insulin-lowering drug, which may be necessary in serious cases. However, reducing your carbohydrate or sugar consumption will naturally lower your insulin levels, insulin resistance and sensitivity to androgens. It will also decrease inflammation and improve your overall health. Even if you are on prescription medication for this condition, most medical professionals will advise you to follow these same recommendations, which usually produce more positive change than the medication itself.

Also, certain vitamins play a key role in insulin stability. For example, Vitamin C decreases cortisol levels and in turn decreases insulin levels. Vitamin D decreases insulin resistance. Magnesium helps to maintain optimal insulin production. Also, exercise is very important as it lowers blood glucose levels.

The takeaway here is this: lowering your insulin levels will correct other hormonal imbalances and help to eliminate your acne.

THYROID

The thyroid is an endocrine gland that not only stores and produces hormones, but is essential for every cell in the body. Thyroid hormones regulate your body's temperature, metabolism, heart rate, and blood pressure and convert food into energy.

Hypothyroidism, or low thyroid levels, result when the thyroid gland does not produce enough thyroid-stimulating hormone (TSH), triiodothyronine (T3) and thyroxine (T4). Hypothyroidism can cause various problems such as fatigue, depression, constipation, weight gain, and skin disorders like acne, cystic acne and dry, thinning hair. Thyroid malfunctions are often due to low levels of iron, selenium, and iron deficiency.

Low thyroid impairs your body's ability to convert beta-carotene into Vitamin A, an important vitamin to maintain skin health and prevent acne. Large doses of Vitamin A can be toxic, so obtain a Vitamin A test to determine if you need to supplement beyond your multivitamin.

Many medications can interfere with thyroid hormones, particularly antibiotics, which more often than not are exactly what the dermatologists prescribe individuals suffering from acne. Toxins and chemicals in our food, home, and work environment disrupt thyroid function as well.

103

Hypothyroidism can also lead to SIBO, which stands for "small intestinal bacterial overgrowth". SIBO occurs when excessive bacteria in the small intestine results in poor nutrient absorption and damage of stomach lining, causing – you guessed it – inflammation. Tired of hearing about poor gut health? If you have any of these symptoms, you may want a thyroid test to check your levels.

TESTOSTERONE/DHT/DHEA

Testosterone is produced by both men and women and is the king of all androgens. Dihydrotestosterone (DHT) is an androgen and chemical derivative of testosterone. DHT controls sebaceous glands and sebum production. Too much testosterone and/or DHT causes skin to become oily, increasing the chances of acne.

Dehydroepiandrosterone (DHEA-S) is another male hormone that the body turns into testosterone. DHEA stimulates oil production, too, and high levels of this hormone will increase the opportunity for acne to occur. Also, the stress hormone cortisol raises DHEA levels, which in turn increases testosterone levels and oil production.

Sex Hormone Binding Globulin (SHBG) is a protein made by the liver that binds to 17 different hormones, including testosterone. Once this happens, the hormone becomes unavailable for use by the body. When these hormones are not bound to SHBG, they are referred to as "free" or 'bioavailable" to be used. If SHBG is too low, there will be more "free" testosterone (too much) that can cause acne breakouts.

Low SHBG levels are caused by excess insulin, insulin resistance and excess androgens. On the other hand, high levels of SHBG can create testosterone deficiency and lead to estrogen dominance that can cause acne as well. Estrogen dominance occurs when a woman has little to no progesterone and has deficient, normal or excessive amounts of estrogen to balance its effects on the body.

Many doctors focus on the "free" testosterone, when, in fact, normalizing SHBG levels should balance the amount of bioavailable testosterone. SHBG levels may be normalized by balancing insulin levels.

There are many strategies to lower high androgen levels without trying to reduce them with medications, including a diet rich in antioxidants such as fruits and vegetables and low in bad carbohydrates and sugars.

Green tea and saw palmetto can be useful in balancing hormones as well. However, I would not try herbs specifically designed to balance hormones or prescription hormone-balancing medications without testing all of these hormones first. Make sure you work with a doctor before taking supplements to adjust your hormones. Self-diagnosing and treating your hormones can have a disastrous effect and completely disrupt your system.

PROGESTERONE/ESTROGEN

Progesterone is a female steroid sex hormone that stimulates the uterus to prepare for pregnancy, regulates menstrual cycles and impacts your libido. Progesterone is a natural androgen blocker, so progesterone deficiency has the potential to cause acne. Some symptoms of low progesterone are low libido, hot flashes, migraines or headaches, depression, anxiety, menstrual-cycle irregularities or cessation of menses.

Estrogen hormones are the primary female hormones responsible for the development and regulation of the female reproductive system. Estradiol, estriol and estrone are three types of estrogen your body makes. Estrogen "turns off" oil production, but the estrogen-acne connection is not that simple. Low progesterone in relation to estrogen, called estrogen dominance, causes acne breakouts, creates weight gain, heavy bleeding, PMS and breast tenderness.

Low thyroid can cause low progesterone that can lead to estrogen dominance, which creates hypothyroidism. The correct progesterone/estrogen balance prevents the conversion of testosterone to DHT that keeps acne away. Also, low progesterone can increase insulin levels that create excess androgens that cause acne. Stress causes our bodies to steal the resources that make progesterone to make stress hormones like cortisol, creating an imbalance or shortage.

Magnesium, B6 and zinc are essential for progesterone production. Low concentrations of these nutrients in our diets, high alcohol consumption, stress, blood-sugar imbalances and some medications like birth control can deplete our bodies of the amounts necessary to carry out important tasks. A PGSN Test or progesterone test can help you determine your levels if you suspect a deficiency.

POLYCYSTIC OVARY SYNDROME

A hormonal disorder, Polycystic Ovary Syndrome (PCOS), affects approximately five to ten percent of women and involves sensitivities to insulin, testosterone and carbohydrates. Some of the signs you may be suffering from PCOS include acne, facial and body hair (not peach fuzz), loss of scalp hair, irregular periods, difficulty becoming pregnant, weight gain despite dieting, and abnormal metabolism. Remember, not every woman will have every symptom and these symptoms do not necessarily mean you have PCOS (consult with your doctor).

There is no one particular test to determine a diagnosis of PCOS, but rather a set of criteria through blood, hormone and ultrasound testing. If you are diagnosed with PCOS, there are medications you can take to lower testosterone and insulin levels. Lifestyle modifications in diet and exercise can help manage PCOS. Limiting processed foods and sugar improves your body's use of insulin and normalizes hormone levels, which can be quite effective, and in my opinion, the best place to start.

HORMONE REPLACEMENT THERAPY

Today Hormone Replacement Therapy (HRT) is more regularly used to balance the body's natural hormone levels. Historically, HRT was used for women experiencing menopause symptoms. Peri-menopause, menopause and post-menopause are often accompanied by fluctuations in estrogen, progesterone and testosterone levels. These fluctuations can create hormonal imbalances.

There are many therapies for bringing balance back to hormones. They can be administered in pills, injections, pellets, and creams. Now men and women are experiencing hormonal imbalances and deficiencies at an earlier age, which I believe is one factor contributing to the rise of adult acne, especially because of one particular hormone replacement that's gained in popularity. Testosterone Replacement Therapy.

TESTOSTERONE REPLACEMENT THERAPY

Testosterone Replacement Therapy (TRT) has become more glamorous and mainstream because of the positive benefits it provides. It helps your body stay leaner, helps retain and build muscle mass, decreases fat, increases sexual desire, helps you sleep better, increases bone density, helps erectile dysfunction, fatigue and depression. Sign me up, right?

However, TRT can cause some side effects such as acne and unwanted hair loss. Be aware some types of birth control pills contain male hormones that can cause and exacerbate existing acne. Hormonal fluctuations and widespread use of HRT may be one of the reasons we are seeing more adult acne cases in women, particularly in their forties, when they never experienced acne in their youth. It is my opinion that the way you eat and your lifestyle exacerbate natural hormone fluctuations creating the need, or illusion of the need, for HRT.

If you have acne, it's a good idea to get your hormones checked. Even if you do not suspect a serious imbalance, it is useful information. It may let you know something is "off" or "out of balance" in your body before you notice anything, allowing you the opportunity to nip it in the bud before it gets worse.

Following this program that recommends an anti-inflammatory diet, detoxing your home and body, taking nutritional supplements, reducing stress, and getting plenty of sleep will help rebalance hormone levels, reducing your acne if not totally curing it.

Only after you have implemented all of these recommendations should you consider hormone replacement if the hormonal problem still persists. This will help you avoid any unnecessary tinkering with your body's delicate systems.

Whether it is through your medical doctor or through a naturopathic doctor, there are specific supplements and bio-identical-hormone prescriptions to adjust hormonal imbalances without using dangerous prescription medications. Do your due diligence and investigate all prescriptions and their potential side effects before you follow what the doctor prescribes.

CHAPTER 10.
Acne Care for Your Skin Type

A combination of dietary and lifestyle modifications with a proper skin-care regimen will provide the best result of success in eliminating your acne. Topical skin-care procedures and products are extremely effective in helping to reduce breakouts, pigmentation and scarring. However, as a stand-alone treatment for chronic or serious acne, skin-care products are not usually successful long term. When deciding which products to buy, you must first identify the variables affecting your acne. Keep in mind, what works well for your friend's acne may be different from what will work well for yours. Acne care is not one-size fits all. What works well for one person may not be best for someone else.

WHAT TYPE OF SKIN DO I HAVE?

Identifying the variables that affect your skin-care regimen success will assist in narrowing down product choices, as well as avoiding wasting money and potentially making your acne worse. Some acne-prone skin types are extremely oily, while other skin types have combination or drier skin types. The category you fall into will dictate how aggressive you can be with your skin-care products.

Acne affects every shade of skin, however, different considerations come into play with different skin colors. It is important to determine if you have a light, medium or dark complexion before you choose which products and treatments will have the least amount of potential side effects

Your age influences how your skin behaves and heals and is another major factor in choosing an effective skin-care regimen. For example, women's skin usually becomes drier after menopause, which tends to make it more sensitive to ingredients and drier climates. On the other hand, during and after menopause, some women (and men too) may use some form of hormone replacement potentially making skin oiler.

Combining aging, hormone replacement and rich/thick anti-aging skin-care formulas will likely result in breakouts.

Sensitive skin, skin that is reactive to many types of ingredients, is becoming more prevalent because of the excessive load of toxins we are breathing, ingesting and putting on our bodies. It is crucial to your success that you are able to identify products that do not irritate and inflame your skin any further. This is why it is not as simple as buying a wash that is labeled "For acne-prone skin."

THE EFFECT OF CLIMATE

The climate (where you live or vacation) influences your skin's moisture levels. Humidity levels influence skin's water or moisture content, which influences the skin's reactions to stripping agents. The higher the humidity level in the air, the better your skin can tolerate dehydrating products. The drier the climate, the less your skin will tolerate multiple stripping agents.

Heat triggers oil production. In hotter climates and in summer months, people tend to have more oily skin. In colder climates and winter months, skin tends to become drier. Turning on your heater at home, at work or in your car reduces moisture levels in the air, and, therefore, in your skin too. This is why there can't be a cookie cutter, one-size-fits-all approach to an acne skin-care regimen. I recommend putting a humidifier in your bedroom during winter months and in drier climates.

OILY, COMBINATION, OR DRY SKIN

There are two different kinds of dry: oil dry (not producing enough oil) and water dry (lack of water, or dehydration). Dehydration means your skin has a water deficiency. These conditions can be caused from internal factors or external factors. Small pores, flakiness, rough patches, wrinkles and inflammation are signs of a lack of oil. Wrinkles, inflammation, and feeling that your skin is tight are signs of dehydration.

Acne sufferers typically buy acne skin-care products that are both oil and water stripping to eliminate the excess oil. You might ask the question, "Isn't that what I am trying to do?' The answer is yes, but not too much. If you are feeling really dry, you need to determine whether your skin-care products are causing this. Too strong or too many drying and dehydrating ingredients in your products will trigger more acne.

What are external factors that cause dryness and dehydration? Skin-care products and weather are two big ones. Any product that contains sodium lauryl sulfate, alcohol, sodium chloride, benzoyl peroxide, salicylic acid, glycolic acid, retinoic acid (Retin- A/tazorac/tretinoin), and other potentially drying ingredients will strip and dehydrate your skin. Stripping the skin is not necessarily bad when you have acne, but when too many of these ingredients are in your skin-care routine it actually makes acne worse. Over-stripping on a regular basis causes the skin to produce more oil to compensate. Also, the more stripped and dehydrated your skin becomes, the greater the irritation.

If your skin becomes too irritated for too long, it becomes inflamed. The result is acne. Often called a reverse breakout, the combination of oil and inflammation creates the very thing you are trying to eliminate. When this happens, dermatologists or skin-care professionals will suggest your skin is just "purging," but most times the products are actually causing it.

The trick or winning combo, which varies for each individual, is to strip the skin just enough to do the job of unclogging pores and killing bacteria while flying under the radar of dehydration and inflammation. So, why do some acne treatments work wonders for some and not for others? Because some people have different levels of water and oil in their skin, are living in different climates that change seasonally, and have different types of sensitivities to ingredients. Additionally, your age and gender also contribute to moisture levels in skin.

For Example:

A typical daily routine begins with a cleanser containing benzoyl peroxide that lathers up and contains some exfoliating beads, followed by a toner containing salicylic acid and alcohol.

Next is a moisturizer that contains a bunch of chemicals used on over-stripped skin with pore-clogging parabens and possibly more acids or BPO's. By the way, these are standard, dermatologist product-combination recommendations for acne patients. Scary!

If your skin is extremely oily, this regimen might be somewhat effective. If you have combination or drier skin, this regimen will cause your skin to become overly sensitive, dry and "peely." It will become red, irritated, uncomfortable, and most likely will result in a reverse breakout because it is too inflamed or you're over moisturizing to alleviate the discomfort. I have seen this scenario in my practice more times than I can count.

My Recommendation: Use no more than one or two stripping agents at a time to avoid the side effects of harsh topicals, and if your skin is more dry with acne, perhaps only one. One of the stripping agents should always include some form of alpha hydroxy acid (AHA), beta hydroxy acid (BHA) or retinoic acid because of the multitude of benefits there are for clearing up acne, post-inflammatory hyperpigmentation, and scarring.

- **For dry skin** – a creamy cleanser twice a day, a low percentage topical retinoid (.025%), AHA or BHA once a day and a light-weight paraben-free moisturizer twice a day

- **For combination skin** – two different cleaners to alternate, one creamy (a.m.), one foaming (p.m.) in addition to your low-percentage topical acid and a light-weight parabens-free moisturizer.

Depending on the acid and its directions, you might be able to use it more than one time per day. If your skin is tolerating the low percentage acid well, you may be able to apply it twice a day. If it is too strong, there will be less room to alter your routine without starting to skip days.

- **For oily skin** – use a foaming cleanser twice per day, in addition to a higher percentage topical acid (retinoid .05%) one time per day and a back-up light-weight paraben-free moisturizer just in case of an emergency.

This means: DO NOT use it every day, twice a day. Only use it when your skin is excessively dry, and then spot treat with moisturizer.

SENSITIVE SKIN

There is no medical definition for sensitive skin. Someone with sensitive or highly reactive skin might get blotchy, itchy or experience a stinging sensation in response to products or weather, or have rosacea, acne or eczema. Sensitive skin could also be caused by your diet (specific foods and additives), and different types of allergens. It is possible these responses may actually be allergic reactions to certain chemical ingredients in your products. It could also be due to using retinoids or alpha/beta hydroxy acids. This may cause some of the same side effects because the acids are too strong (too high a percentage), or there are too many stripping or dehydrating ingredients in your regimen.

If you are getting rashes, redness or inflammation, stop using the product. Mild dryness and flaking are normal reactions to AHA/BHA. If you are experiencing mild irritation using AHA/BHA/retinoids, cut back on the dosage or reduce the effectiveness by combining it with moisturizer to see if that helps alleviate the problem.

Once your protective barrier is compromised, you will need to let it settle down and heal for a few days before you try the retinoid/alpha hydroxy acid again. This is also why I recommend limiting multiple stripping ingredients so as to avoid compromising your skin. Doing so will increase the skin's tolerance to these acids and allow you to reap their anti-acne and anti-aging benefits.

If you think you have "sensitive" skin, here is a list of ingredients to steer clear of: artificial fragrances, food allergens, parabens, lanolin, sulfates, chemicals you cannot pronounce, alcohol (internal and external), retinoids and alpha/beta hydroxyl acids in high percentages. Also avoid extreme hot or cold water, scrubs, and layering too many products or using too many stripping skin-care products.

DARKER SKIN

Darker skin tones describe a range of skin colors from black to brown, olive to yellow, or tanned white skin. The causes of acne in skin of color (SOC) are the same as in light-skinned people. However, SOC is more susceptible to acne because it tends to have more sebaceous glands that are larger and produce more oil. It also typically has more skin shedding, which increases the likelihood of clogged pores. SOC also has larger, more active melanocytes and a stronger inflammatory reaction that increases the opportunity for a breakout and post-inflammatory hyperpigmentation (PIH).

Exfoliating agents such as professional chemical peels, enzymes and at-home skin-care treatments are a great option in treating acne for all skin colors, especially darker skin tones. Most quasi-medical or laser treatments are too invasive for SOC and don't really work well for acne in general. Treating SOC with chemical peels without a pre- and post-treatment regimen, and chemical peels that are too deep or done too frequently can potentially cause hyperpigmentation (brown spots) or hypopigmentation (white spots).

The darker you are, the more prone you are to PIH. PIH can also be caused by acne/pimples, burns, scratches, excessive dryness and other minor skin traumas, as well as chemical peels and different types of lasers. No matter what your skin color is, always start conservatively with any skin-care treatment or product. It is easier to increase the strength gradually than to begin too aggressively and have to reverse PIH.

My Recommendation: Prepping with a pre-home care regimen before a peel is an absolute must for skin of color. Gradually and gently preparing the skin will give it time to adjust and avoid post-peel complications. A gentle wash with a low percentage alpha hydroxy acid and an SPF are all that is needed.

Occasionally I recommend skin lighteners too, depending upon the severity of acne and PIH. However, lightening agents, especially those containing prescription and non-prescription hydroquinone (HQ), can contain thick, pore-clogging ingredients that provoke acne.

Rather than over-exposing skin with a high-percentage chemical peel, I suggest starting with progressive peels. Progressive peels are superficial and do not cause immediate exfoliation. They are also good for preparing for more aggressive, mid-depth peels with mild sloughing. Progressive peels are usually performed every two weeks, but I advise once a month in SOC to avoid over-stimulating the skin and potentially causing PIH.

I always send my clients home with 1% over-the–counter (OTC) hydrocortisone lotion to apply post-peel three to five days as an insurance policy against PIH. It helps to reduce inflammation, which can trigger PIH and acne breakouts. It also makes for a good spot treatment for acne.

NOTE: Whether HQ, also known as bleaching cream, is safe for the skin is a serious debate. Over time, HQ can become less effective and cause ochronosis (skin darkening), especially in SOC. Although rare, I do recommend 2% HQ in my practice, but never as a long-term indefinite part of anyone's, especially SOC clients, skin-care routine. I use other more "natural" lightening agents that typically take longer to see results, but are safer and tend to be longer lasting.

Hydrocortisone (not the OTC ones at the drug store) is not to be used for long periods of time. It can thin the skin and exacerbate skin disorders like acne, rosacea, and perioral dermatitis. With mild, progressive peels, this light, cosmeceutical formula of hydrocortisone can sometimes double as a moisturizer and temporarily help hydrate post-peel dry and acne-prone skin.

ADULT AND AGING SKIN

Why am I'm getting wrinkles and pimples? Actually, it is not uncommon to be simultaneously battling aging skin and breakouts. Clinical studies indicate adult acne is on the rise, with up to 55% of the adult population between 20 to 40 years of age being diagnosed with acne. Adult acne is more common in women than in men. The higher rates among women are likely due to:

- **Fluctuating hormones** – Fluctuating hormone levels can be caused by going on birth control pills, going off birth control pills, changing types of birth control, use of bio-identical hormones, menstrual periods, pregnancy, breast feeding, peri-menopause, and menopause. Whew!

- **Medication side effects** – Nearly 60% of Americans take prescription drugs; half of them are on least two prescription medications and 20% of them at least five! Statistically speaking, the older a person gets, the more prescription drugs they are prescribed. Women are prescribed more drugs than men. Antibiotics and antidepressants are the top two drugs prescribed in the US. If you think they are safe and don't have side effects, think again. One of the potential side effects of prescription medications is acne.

- **Stress** – You have already read how stress can trigger acne. The older we get, the more stress we are exposed to physically, emotionally and mentally.

- **Garbage Products** – Garbage skin-care products full of synthetic, harsh, toxic, pore- clogging ingredients that are harmful for your skin.

- **Food and Diet** – Poor food quality and lack of nutrients multiplied by years of living on Earth, exposed to all the factors above, equal premature aging and acne.

The older men and women become, the more we notice our "imperfections" and start buying and experimenting with products that are "anti-aging." Products labeled "anti-aging" tend to be richer and more emollient. This can increase the likelihood of a breakout in adults with oily and combination skin types.

Although older men and postmenopausal women tend to have drier and more sensitive skin, many women have oily skin naturally and do not need thick anti-aging serums and creams. Even if your skin feels dry, it might be dehydrated, not oil-dry; it may be due to your diet, lack of water, over-stripping product choices or climate.

My Recommendation: Be cautious when buying a product labeled as anti-aging when you have oil- or acne-prone skin. Anti-aging products often contain anti-oxidants such as Vitamins C and E, which can be great for normal and dry skin, but trigger breakouts in oily or combination skin.

In acne-prone or sensitive skin types, Vitamin C can cause redness and irritation too. Vitamin E used topically is reserved for people with dry skin/low amounts of oil. For obvious reasons, applying oil to oily skin can backfire. Be aware that many skin-care companies state their anti-aging formulas are safe for combination and acne-prone skin. I say, "When in doubt, skip it"! Consuming antioxidants, taking your supplements and following an anti-inflammatory diet will benefit aging and acne-prone skin more than applying antioxidants topically.

The good news is that many ingredients in acne products are also anti-aging. Using glycolic, salicylic and/or retinoic acid in the right percentage and formulation help diminish breakouts and reduce scarring. The same ingredients aid in improving the appearance of fine lines and wrinkles by stimulating collagen production. They also help to fade brown spots and keep skin smoother and brighter.

TEEN SKIN

Oilier skin and hair are brought on by the hormonal changes of puberty. Any age group can experience acne, however, when androgens/male hormones surge during adolescence, pregnancy, or starting/stopping birth control pills, breakouts become more likely.

For example, teen acne can be dealt with much the same as adult acne. I deal with teen-acne clients the same way I do my adult-acne clients. I provide them basic information on the factors that can exacerbate their acne, dietary and lifestyle changes, basic and simple skin-care product recommendations and recommend clinical facials if necessary.

My Recommendation: For teens with severe acne where scarring is beginning to occur, I recommend seeing a dermatologist who might prescribe medications temporarily to stop any further scarring. These prescription medications should not be taken long term. Instead, they should be used as a way to reduce the acne and scarring in the short term while you have time to modify your diet and lifestyle and implement your new product and treatment regimen.

People, let alone teenagers in particular, have a difficult time changing their eating habits, but their health and acne resolution depend on it. If what you eat and lifestyle changes are not made, as soon as you stop taking your prescription medication, your acne usually comes back. Medication does not cure acne; at best, it just helps to control it. The long-term effects of prescription medication are bad for skin, and in teenagers who are still developing, it can really impact their health.

NOTE: Do not let your dermatologist keep your child on antibiotics in addition to other medications indefinitely. The doctor should have a clear plan of how long medication should be taken. If not, RUN! If you do not see results in the amount of time recommended, quit. It is not working. Also remember, BCP's are not without side effects either.

CHAPTER 11.
What Products Should I Use?

Whether it's acne or another skin condition, it's always a good idea to keep your skin-care routine clean, clinical and minimal. Whenever possible, seek professional advice and use clinical products.

Clinical products are formulated with more concentrated ingredients and better technology. Unfortunately, not all clinical products are "green", but cosmeceutical lines tend to be much cleaner than over-the-counter and prescription skin-care formulas. This typically means higher quality ingredients, no parabens, no dyes, and no artificial fragrances.

My Recommendation: Too many layers of product weigh down the skin and have the potential to clog pores even when using non-comedogenic products (products specifically formulated not to clog pores). Keep your product use to a minimum to reduce the chances of breaking out. Save your time and money, and do not let the media or fear of aging coax you into buying unnecessary products because you have been told you need them.

DO: Morning routine

1. Use a gentle cleanser wash.
2. Use a scrub, only if necessary (see "Scrubs" in the "Products" section).
3. Ice your face.
4. Use a hyaluronic serum or light moisturizer if needed (see "Moisturizers" in the "Products" section).
5. Use sunscreen (only if plans include being outside for an extended period).
6. Use makeup if you choose.

DON'T: Do not apply moisturizer, sunblock, and makeup as three separate products. This is like putting on three coats or three moisturizers; only apply two at the most.

For example, use moisturizer and makeup, or sunblock and makeup. Some foundations called BB cream (beauty balm) contain moisturizer and sunblock in a tinted cream. This is one way to get all three in one layer, but make sure it's a mineral makeup formulated for oily and acne-prone skin.

DO: Evening routine

1. Use a gentle cleanser or mild, foaming cleanser
2. Maybe use a scrub (only if not used in the morning routine).
3. Ice your face.
4. Use AHA, BHA or Retin-A product (serum form if possible).
5. Use a light moisturizer (only if necessary).

CLEANSERS

I recommend having two different kinds of cleansers: one gentle, non-lathering creamy cleanser and one mild, foaming sulfate-free cleanser for problematic skin. Your skin's condition will dictate which cleanser will be more effective at certain times versus others. For example, how oily your skin is, how much you are working out, if you wear makeup, if it's hot or cold, humid or dry, what other products you are using in combination with it, or if you just had a facial or chemical peel, which requires gentler aftercare.

Gentle cleansers should not over-strip or dehydrate, allowing the skin to tolerate AHAs, BHAs, or retinoids much more easily. They should also be gentle enough to use post peeling. Gentle cleansers are great for drier climates, combination and sensitive skin or for days when you are heavy handed with your acne treatment and over-dry your skin. A mild foaming cleanser is also great for problematic skin because it usually contains a salicylic or glycolic acid in a low percentage to provide a deeper pore cleansing. This comes in handy, especially at the end of the day, when your skin has built up more dirt, oil or makeup.

The oil cleansing method is very popular right now for washing oily and acne-prone skin types. This method can seem great at first because when skin is dried out and irritated the oil is calming, hydrating and soothing. However, after a few days of oil cleansing, the skin becomes well hydrated and no longer needs the moisturizing benefit and may start to break out again. Scrubs and AHA's help to balance oil cleansing, assuming the type and formulation of the cleanser is just right, but even then, it's risky.

My Recommendation: I think it's better to skip the oil- cleansing method and instead practice a gentler routine to eliminate the risk of breaking out entirely. However, if you intend to try this method, do so only once each day maximum and use an exfoliant of some kind (a must!).

TONERS

In theory, with a good skin-care routine and products one should not need a toner. However that is not always the case. I personally like toners as long as you get the right one. The right one depends on how oily your skin is and what else you are using. After cleansing, toners can help remove excess oil, dirt, makeup and sunscreen. However depending on what is in the toner, it could dry out, irritate or add too much moisture to your skin.

On the other hand, if you are in between needing one and two stripping agents, a toner may just give your skin the boost you need without being too harsh. It is also great for after shaving, pre/post workout, or for skin that doesn't tolerate low-percentage acid serums well. They key is choosing the right one.

My Recommendation: Look for toners that contain hyaluronic acid, salicylic acid and maybe tocopheryl acetate (Vitamin E) depending on how dry your skin is (better would be depending on the dryness of your skin). Avoid toners that contain alcohol because they strip and break down the skin's barrier. Avoid cetyl alcohol and stearyl alcohol because these are emollients that moisturizer skin. Avoid petroleum in toner because it forms a film on your face that blocks your skin from breathing. Avoid sodium laureth sulfate because it will dry out your skin.

SCRUBS

Some experts say "yes" to scrubs for acne, some say "no." I say it all depends on the situation. In a perfect world, results are better if you utilize both mechanical and chemical exfoliation. Physically removing buildup in textured, coarse skin or problematic acne-prone skin helps remove excess dead skin (potentially pore clogging) and allows other products to penetrate more effectively. You want to limit scrubbing to only a few times per week and never on irritated, overly dry or inflamed skin.

My Recommendation: Do not over scrub, meaning either too harshly or too often. Avoid nut scrubs like apricot and walnut as well as coconut and oatmeal fibers. These kinds of scrubs can cause microscopic lacerations in your skin.

Do not use loofahs, buff sponges, washcloths or electronic scrub brushes as a type of scrub or in combination with your scrub. Loofah, buff sponges and washcloths can breed bacteria and be too abrasive. I have found that electronic or sonic scrub brushes usually make acne worse, even the ones that state they are good for acne; just avoid them for now.

Scrub brushes or sonic waves stimulate oil glands and amplify the drying effect of your acne products, creating too much irritation and inflammation. Use a scrub that does not contain other drying agents such as emulsifying ingredients or is high lathering (creates bubbles). Go for polyethylene beads, jojoba beads or diatomaceous earth, to name a few.

ACIDS

Glycolic (AHA), salicylic (BHA) and retinoic acids fight acne, reduce scarring and lighten dark spots. The level or strength of the acid depends upon whether it is over the counter (OTC), cosmeceutical or prescription. Be cautious using prescription Retin-A's/Tazorac/tretinoin because they are stronger and can count as two stripping agents in one. Even OTC acids can be too harsh.

If you need to go the dermatologist route, always request the lowest strength retinoid, AHA or BHA to get started and increase the prescription if needed. Also, do not use harsh cleansing or stripping agents with prescription retinoids in the beginning to avoid creating more acne. If your prescription is too harsh causing dry, red, irritated or peely skin, you won't use it as often, and for acids to be most effective, your skin needs a consistent daily dose to prevent and clear up breakouts.

Benzoyl peroxide (BPO) is not an acid, but I am including it in the exfoliating section because it induces flaking and dryness like glycolics, retinols and salicylates do. BPO penetrates into the follicle and kills bacteria versus unclogging the pores in the way acids do. BPO can be extremely irritating because it is often too strong/too high a percentage or is being used in combination with other harsh ingredients/products.

Also many BPO formulations, if they are not micronized molecules, are too large to get down deep into the pore to kill bacteria. Instead the BPO sits on top of the skin where it causes burning, inflammation and excessive dryness.

My Recommendation: Prescription "acid" formulas come in either a gel, lotion or cream formula. Choose a gel or lotion to avoid exposure to thick, pore-clogging agents. If you are going to try to use a BPO, use a gentle, cream cleanser formula once each morning, so you can continue to use your acids without risk of irritation and over-drying. A BPO in a low percentage, ideally 2.5% and no more than 5%, is good.

MOISTURIZERS

Many people and experts believe that we need to use a moisturizer every day. Moisturizer is not necessarily to be used routinely, but rather determined on a case-by-case basis. If you do not feel dry, you do not need moisturizer. If your skin feels dry, tight or flakey, it is likely due to your skin-care regimen. This is why I have previously recommended limiting your use of stripping and dehydrating products. They will cause your skin distress, transdermal water loss and create the need for moisturizer. Lastly, if your skin is oily, you have nature's moisturizer!

It is, however, a good idea to have an appropriate moisturizer as a backup in your clear-skin regimen. This is for those days when your skin gets a little too dried out because you over-exfoliated, had a chemical peel or maybe your skin was subjected to harsh weather. You can also spot treat moisturizer by only applying it where your face is dry.

Eye cream is another story. The skin under the eyes is much thinner and does not contain oil glands to keep it lubricated like the skin on the rest of your face.

Now the million-dollar question: Which moisturizer? There are three different properties in moisturizers. They are occlusive, humectant and emollient.

Occlusive moisturizers physically block trans-epidermal water loss (TEWL). Some common occlusive ingredients include mineral oil, lanolin, petrolatum, paraffin and silicone derivatives that give them that "thick" or "greasy" texture.

Emollient moisturizers help to smooth and hydrate skin with oil. Some common emollient ingredients include dimethicone, castor oil, isopropyl isosterate, octyl stearate, and propylene glycol.

Humectant moisturizers help to hydrate skin by attracting water. Some common humectant ingredients include hyaluronic acid, urea, ammonium and sodium lactate, sorbitol and glycerin. Too much glycerin in a formula can give it that sticky texture. Some moisturizers can contain one or more of these moisturizing properties. For example, it may contain both emollient and humectant ingredients. Other ingredients commonly added to moisturizers for their anti-inflammatory benefits include aloe vera, green tea, allantoin, zinc and copper.

My Recommendation: Finding the perfect moisturizer will be the most difficult aspect of choosing skin-care products. Unfortunately, without seeing your face, I cannot choose one for you or give you a blanket recommendation. What I can tell you is to never use occlusive moisturizers. Avoid emollient moisturizers when possible and try to stick to humectant moisturizers.

Avoid eye creams that are too thick because they can migrate down past the eye area and clog your pores. I recommend gel and light-weight eye cream formulas. Do not apply an emollient moisturizer if you are going to be following it with sunblock and/or liquid foundation. This would be like wearing three moisturizers. The fewer layers of product on your skin, the less likely it is that a breakout will occur.

NOTE: There are quite a few studies that suggest moisturizing may offer temporary relief, but may be harmful to the natural hydration process. Your skin can start to become "dependent" on outside sources of moisture rather than manufacturing its own.

SUNSCREENS

There are two types of sunscreen (SPF): physical and chemical. Physical sunscreens block the sun's rays and contain zinc oxide or titanium oxide. On the positive side, physical sunscreens provide a physical barrier for the skin, outperform chemical blocks, last longer on the skin and are considered less toxic. On the negative side, they can be pore clogging, feel thick and look white on the skin.

Chemical sunscreens absorb the sun's rays. A few of the popular chemical sunblock agents include Paba, Avobenzone, or Dioxybenzone. On the positive side, chemical sunscreens can be lightweight and potentially non-pore clogging. On the negative side, chemical sunscreens are less effective than physical blocks, protect skin a shorter amount of time, have many safety concerns, contain a lot of skin-irritating chemicals and can still be pore clogging.

NOTE: Keep in mind, there is no SPF past 50. Anything claiming to be greater than 50 SPF is creative marketing. If you spend any extended length of time outside in direct sunlight, there is no sunblock out there that will protect you enough. You will need a hat (wide-brimmed – not a baseball cap) and appropriate coverage with clothing for maximum protection.

I am probably going to be criticized for this, but if you predominantly work indoors, daily sunblock isn't necessary. That's right, I said it. Sunblock is notorious for causing acne breakouts and skin irritation. Even sunblock that is "specially formulated for oily or acne-prone skin" can cause breakouts. Many of the ingredients in sunblocks are toxic and cause all kinds of allergic reactions, especially on already inflamed and compromised skin. If you wear makeup/foundation/powder, it is possible it contains some level of SPF in it.

If you must wear sunblock because you are going hiking, doing yard work, or are at the beach, then yes to the sunblock. In addition to the sunblock, you will need a brimmed, sun-protective hat, because no sunblock can totally protect your skin from hours of sun exposure.

MAKEUP

Makeup can cause or exacerbate acne. However, if you have had acne for years, it is not likely the makeup is the sole cause of it. Many ingredients and toxic chemicals in your makeup can clog pores and increase inflammation in the skin, which can result in more breakouts, redness and hyperpigmentation. Makeup labeled "non-comedogenic" or "oil-free" does not guarantee it will not clog your pores or cause breakouts. People with oily skin have larger pores. The weight of using too many layers of products or makeup that is too heavy will cause it to get into the pores. This can block oil from coming out of the follicle freely, potentially creating blackheads and breakouts.

My Recommendation: Mineral makeup is the best choice next to abstinence. Loose mineral powder is the safest bet. Sometimes, my acne clients complain that mineral makeup does not have good coverage. This is sometimes true but, at some point, you are going to have to compromise if you want your breakouts to minimize. Where can I find this makeup? Find an aesthetician, medi-spa, cosmetic surgeon's office or cosmetic store specializing in green products that carries quality, mineral makeup with more coverage.

NOTE: Many cosmetic companies started adding minerals to their makeup and calling it "mineral makeup." It is only a marketing ploy. However, mineral makeup is supposed to be non-toxic, non-chemical and non-acne promoting, which is not always the case. Keep in mind that just because a product is listed as natural, green or organic does not mean that it doesn't contain potentially pore-clogging ingredients for acne-prone skin types (refer to "Additional Resources"). It may be intended for dry, non-acne-prone skin that needs the moisturizing properties. Make sure the mineral makeup also states it is for oily or combination skin. Drier and sensitive skin types should also use mineral makeup because it does not contain the harsh irritating chemicals.

CHAPTER 12.
At Home Tips

SHAVING

Shaving correctly is imperative for men who are prone to acne and raised bumps. If possible, do not shave every day to avoid constant skin aggravation. Use an electric shaver or a single- blade manual razor when possible instead of multi-bladed razors. Multi-bladed razors utilize one blade to push the skin away from the hair allowing the other blades to get in for a closer shave. In this way, hair is cut below the skin surface causing irritation and possible ingrown hairs. Pulling your skin taut will increase the chance of cutting the hair too short as well.

Rinse your blade between shaving strokes to eliminate having to redo areas. This will help alleviate unnecessary irritation. Never shave dry. Pre-shave oil can help prep the skin to avoid nicks and razor burn. However, depending on how it has been formulated, it can also pose a potential acne risk. It's always a good idea to ice after shaving for its skin-calming effects, as described more in the following section.

ICING

Icing your skin is the best-kept secret in combating acne. It reduces swelling around the follicle and sebaceous glands and allows for better absorption of product. It can be as simple as filling a small plastic bag with ice and applying it for ten minutes twice a day during your skin-care routine (ideal), but even one time per day for five minutes is better than nothing. The point is to do it. If you are busy, get an ice mask that has Velcro so you can be hands-free. Make sure you choose a mask that also covers the sides of the face enough to be effective around your jawline and neck.

My Recommendation: I would start by icing twice a day after you wash your face and before you put on any toners or serums. If you can find more time to ice, go for it.

EXTRACTIONS

The problem with extractions is that most people aren't doing them correctly. Some mistakes include trying to extract blemishes that are not "ripe" or "ready" for extraction, not properly prepping the skin, using nails that are long or sharp, over-squeezing or picking the blemish or applying too many drying agents on blemishes and causing scabs.

Also, attempting too many extractions can cause follicles to swell. Swollen follicles can bump against the neighboring follicles and cause a constriction. This constriction can obstruct the natural flow of oil and skin shedding creating a blockage, inflammation, bacterial invasion and formation of another pimple. This in turn bumps into the next follicle causing another obstruction and swelling and then bumps into another and another. This is how acne can spread like wildfire!

My Recommendation: If you want to extract a blemish or blackhead, you first have to make sure your nails are short, your hands and face are washed, you have exfoliated, your face is steamed and that you only extract blackheads or whiteheads. Do not extract closed comedones (closed whiteheads), cystic acne, or pimples/pustules that do not have a whitehead on them. Stop extracting if it doesn't come out easily.

CHAPTER 13.
Acne No-Nos

The following list is provided as a summary of how to most effectively take care of your acne-prone skin:

Say no to:

- **products with artificial fragrances, dyes, sulfates, phthalates or parabens**

- **oil cleansing**
  It is just too risky; skip it.

- **face wipes and makeup removers**
  Makeup removers should only be needed to take off waterproof mascara.

- **waterproof mascara**

- **over-washing your skin**

  Wash no more than two times per day on average and never go to bed without washing your makeup off.

- **picking pimples that are not ready**

- **picking and peeling dry skin or flakes**

- **electronic scrub brushes**

  They stimulate oil production and drive already stripping/dehydrating acne products further into the follicles causing increased inflammation.

- **too many stripping ingredients and products**

  Use only one or two stripping products in your home routine at most, depending on all the previously mentioned variables.

- **too many layers of products on the face**

  Less is more no matter how good the quality of products.

- **over-moisturizing**

- **primers**

  No heavy foundations either.

- **chemical sunscreens**
  Be discerning of physical sunscreens.

- **waxing or shaving the face** (if you're a woman)
  If you are a man, do not shave if you do not have to. If you can, choose an electric razor over a double-edged razor. If you have to use a razor, use a single blade.

- **dermaplaning**
  It irritates acne-prone skin and can cause a breakout.

- **department-store advice and self-prescribing**
  Do not rely on your local department store, your best friend, the Internet, a magazine or television for your skin-care advice.

- **spa facials**
  They feel nice but usually cause breakouts. Only clinical facials.

- **cortisone injections for cystic acne**
  The potential for scarring is devastating and usually doesn't show up until a year or so later. Avoid it if you can.

- **micro-needling**

  If you have active acne, micro-needling causes too much inflammation and trauma to your skin, increasing risk for breakouts. You must wait to be acne-free. No home rollers/home micro-needling, as you can tear your skin easily.

- **laser treatments**

  If you have active acne, light therapy is okay, but no laser resurfacing or fraxel whatsoever. They cause too much inflammation and trauma. The potential for hyperpigmentation and more breakouts is way too high. Darker skin tones should never have laser therapy.

CHAPTER 14.
Professional Acne Treatments

There are many benefits to working with an aesthetician/skin-care specialist and using professional products. The odds of clearing your acne will be much higher using an aesthetician than self-prescribing via Internet, drugstore or department store. Aestheticians working in spas and salons typically perform your superficial, relaxing, spa-type facials. Do not get facials from these types of aestheticians. Not only will it not help your acne, but most likely it will make it worse. Spa facials have their place in skin-care, just not with clearing acne.

HOW DO I FIND A CLINICAL AESTHETICIAN?

Trying to address skin-care problems on your own can be very frustrating. If you have acne, seeking professional advice will produce faster results and save you a lot of money. Clinical aestheticians have a higher level of education and training allowing them to provide deeper cleansing and exfoliation methods through specialized products and procedures designed for corrective treatment and visible results. Typically you find clinical aestheticans working in medi-spas and occasionally, like me, working on their own after years of working with doctors.

Schedule a consultation with a clinical aesthetician/skin clinic to discuss your current regimen and products used and formulate a plan going forward. If your acne is severe, see a dermatologist as well.

Where can you find a good aesthetician? Start your search by looking for clinical or medical aestheticians on YELP or Google. Doctor's offices and medi-spas are a good start, but tend to be more expensive. There are some great aestheticians that work on their own that can provide clinical skin-care too. You might want to get personal referrals, but make sure it's from someone being treated for acne. Just because a skin-care provider is good at their craft does not mean they specialize in acne. They will be able to discuss your current skin-care regimen in detail and formulate a plan going forward. If your acne is severe, see a dermatologist as well.

I have created a list of suggestions for questions to ask when deciding on an aesthetician. You don't have to ask all the questions, but this list is a good place to start.

QUESTIONS TO ASK AN AESTHETICIAN

- What are their credentials?

- How long have they been in practice?

- What product lines do they use?

- Does the aesthetician do their own consultations and do they charge for them?

  NOTE: The answer should be yes to both, doing their own consult and charging for it. Many medi-spa facilities and doctor's offices have one person (the sales person) do the initial consult and sell the product/services and another person to perform the service. The same person should be recommending and administering your products and treatments throughout the entire process.

I charge for my consultations because my years of training and extensive experience have enabled me to fine- tune and condense that knowledge and pass it on to the client. Even if you do not opt for treatment with me, you will leave with all kinds of useful recommendations and priceless advice that alone could help you clear your acne.

- Do they specialize in acne?

- Do they have experience with ethnic skin? (If you have it.)

- Do they have a website for you to read about their philosophy on acne and skin-care?

- Are you comfortable when you arrive at your appointment? How are you greeted?
  NOTE: It is important to listen to your gut, especially when people are going to be poking and prodding at your skin. Are they warm and friendly or are you just another number? Does the place look clean?

- What does the aesthetician look like? Does their skin appear healthy?
  NOTE: Clearly you're not going to take advice from someone with acne. In general, aestheticians should be a walking billboard for what they preach and practice.

- When you meet the aesthetician, do they listen to you?
  NOTE: They should listen and ask you questions about what skin-care products you are using topically, what your diet is, what lifestyle habits may be contributing to your acne, and what you have already tried that has or has not worked for you.

- Do they try to push you to do treatments you are not comfortable with?

  NOTE: You should always make sure that the course of treatment you decide on makes sense to you and is one you are open to pursuing. Also, they should not recommend starting with the most aggressive treatment option unless you have already tried lesser aggressive options without success.

- Do they prepare you for all the possible side effects and potential down time of the treatments or products they recommend so you are informed of the process?

- Do they recognize when your acne condition is complicated and recommend a dermatologist to work in conjunction with you?

- Do they make promises your acne will go away if you do the treatments and buy the products they say?

  NOTE: No one should make guarantees or promises that a product or procedure will cure your acne. This sets unrealistic expectations. As we know, chronic acne has to be treated from the inside out and outside in.

There are great aestheticians out there. After doing your research, book a couple of consults with your top choices and bring the list of questions to each appointment. At the end of the consult, if you're not completely comfortable with the aesthetician for whatever reason, keep looking. Just because someone is a doctor or trained in skin-care does not always make them a good fit for you. I know it can be hard suffering with acne, but do not let it cause you to obtain treatment or services from someone you are not excited about.

CLINICAL SKIN-CARE PRODUCTS

Clinical aestheticians use professional skin-care products usually cosmeceutical and occasionally pharmaceutical grade.

Cosmeceutical refers to cosmetic products with active ingredients that have medical or drug-like benefits that are known to be beneficial in some way.

Pharmaceutical skin-care products have ingredients classified by the FDA as drugs. Neither one of these types of skin-care products are available over the counter because they contain higher concentrations of active ingredients, are higher quality and are targeted to treat specific skin conditions. Professional skin-care products are obtained through licensed aestheticians, medi-spas and doctor's offices.

Quality products and a proper home-care routine can make or break your success in achieving great skin. Even though clinical skin-care products are used "at home", they should still be considered a professional acne treatment. What you do every day makes the biggest difference in your skin, for better or worse.

NOTE: If your clinical aesthetician is trying to send you home with seven different new products that cost $1,000, move on to another facility. If you have a budget, your aesthetician can help you prioritize products that will support the treatment you're receiving. Remember, less is more with acne-prone skin. Start with less and if you need to add additional products, do so later after your skin has adjusted to the new products.

CLINICAL FACIALS

Clinical facials are designed to treat problematic skin versus a traditional spa facial that is designed for basic cleansing, hydration and relaxation. Clinical facials utilize the proper tools and concentrated, active products designed to make a visible difference or change in the skin. Clinical facials have a specific-treatment protocol based on your individual needs versus a spa facial with a cookie-cutter protocol. Usually, but not always, they are performed in medi-spas and cosmetic doctors' offices.

I am always surprised when I find out my client's dermatologist's office does not offer clinical/medical facials, but rather only oral and topical prescription drugs and over-the-counter home-care products. A regimen of clinical facials goes hand in hand with prescription medications when clearing acne.

Clinical or medical facials include cleansing, exfoliating, extractions and hydrating, but on a more intense level than a spa facial or classic European facial. Expect these extractions to be unpleasant or downright painful. Medical facials may include some light therapy, high-frequency or hyperbaric oxygen to reduce inflammation and kill bacteria.

Exfoliation can be accomplished using gentle enzymes, a chemical peel or both to lift dead skin cells, brighten and smooth skin. Chemical peels combined with a medical facial are far more effective than peels alone. Cleaning your pores with extractions and removing the dead skin by exfoliating first allows the peel to penetrate more evenly and effectively. Your skin type and severity of acne are both factors in determining the frequency and level of medical facials.

My Recommendation: Clients with many extractions often need to come in every two weeks initially, then transition to monthly clinical facials.

CHEMICAL PEELS

Chemical peels can be the safest, most effective and least expensive treatment to help clear acne. Peels do everything your topical home acid does, but stronger. They help prevent and clear acne, diminish discoloration, stimulate collagen (great for fine lines, wrinkles and scars) and help brighten and smooth the skin's surface. Chemical peels, whether light (mild) or mid-depth, along with a home-care regimen, aid in clearing up acne, minimize scarring and discoloration throughout the process.

Downtime for a chemical peel is very subjective. In general, medical facials I administer are considered "no downtime," meaning you may experience blotchy skin for the rest of the day and light flaking for the following week. Stronger peels create more shedding that may be considered noticeable (more downtime, based on your tolerance and comfort). Always ask what type of acid, what percentage of acid and how many applications per treatment they plan on using if you are concerned.

NOTE: Every peel you try may be different, even if the same type of acid in the same percentage is used by the same aesthetician. Never assume from one aesthetician to the next that your chemical peel will have the same amount of downtime as the last one. This is due to the different variables at any given time that can be affecting how your peel turns out.

For example:

- where you live
- the time of year
- your gender and the time of month
- other products used with the peel
- other products being used at home (Are they the same or different than before?)
- over-the-counter or prescription medications you are or were using during the peel process
- your stress level.

LEVULAN/PHOTODYNAMIC THERAPY

Levulan or Photodynamic Therapy (PDT) is safe, non-laser light that is used in conjunction with levulinic acid in a two-part process to selectively target keratosis and sebaceous glands. The blue light activates the Levulan, shrinking the tissues and sebaceous glands to decrease acne. It is typical to experience significant reddening, swelling and peeling following treatment.

The degree to which the patient experiences these side effects depends on how long the solution was allowed to sit on the skin's surface and how long the blue light was used to activate the solution. Sometimes IPL (intensed pulsed light) is used to activate the Levulan. I do not recommend skins of color use this method because of the risk of burns and hyperpigmentation caused by the IPL. Expect at least a seven to ten day recovery. PDT is helpful in reducing acne; however, it usually takes more than one treatment, can be quite expensive and often comes back.

OTHER DEVICES

Non-invasive acne-clearing devices include, but are not limited to, blue, LED (Light Emitting Diode), high-frequency and electronic heat. These machines are all designed to destroy bacteria inside the follicle. As a stand- alone treatment, whether FDA approved or not, it will not cure your acne.

If you have the extra money and time, it may be somewhat helpful as an adjunctive tool in your clinical aesthetician's office, but will only have minimal benefits at best. As for buying over-the-counter devices, forget about it.

CHAPTER 15.
Treatments for Acne Scars

There are several treatments that can work well for acne scarring depending on the type and severity of scars, your skin tone and your budget. Scarring is difficult to fully eliminate. Expectations need to be realistic. A good result for scars is when they become less noticeable and skin is softer and smoother.

Depending on State regulations, certified aestheticians or doctors' offices can perform treatment on scars. Investigate within your community who has the most experience and best reputation for each treatment you may be considering. Make sure they are known and specialize in acne scarring. Always do **at least two** different consults and check before receiving treatment to make sure they do not have any medical complaints if they are doing more invasive laser resurfacing.

NOTE: Read their reviews in online platforms specific to the service you are looking into. They may have fabulous reviews for breast augmentations and liposuction, which has nothing to do with lasers and acne scarring. If you are thinking of a laser procedure for your acne scarring, investigate who will be doing your laser treatment. Your results will depend on how much experience this individual has with acne scar revision in general and with the particular method they will use.

MEDICAL PEELS

Medical peels for scarring? Yes! Absolutely! Assuming all your bases are covered: right strength/percentage of acid matched to the appropriate skin type with the proper home-care routine. Once acne is alleviated, a mid-depth or medical strength chemical peel is great for addressing scarring and remaining discoloration. Trichloroacetic acid (TCA) peels are great options for mid-depth. Around seven to ten days downtime should be expected to play it on the safe side.

My Recommendation: Start with progressive peels before trying a medical peel. Begin with the least invasive treatment and work your way to stronger treatments as needed. Also, if you want your treatments to be successful, you have to have proper home-care products. It is just as important to spend your money on a good home-care regimen as it is to spend it on medical treatments if you have to choose.

The products will cost more money than over-the-counter choices, but a skin clinic should be able to offer you reasonably priced products. If the cost of professional products is a concern, keep in mind that you typically wind up spending more on over-the-counter products that don't work than if you had purchased three really good professional products that do.

MICRO-NEEDLING AND PLATELET-RICH PLASMA

Micro-Needling (aka Collagen Induction Therapy [CIT]) and Platelet-Rich Plasma (PRP, aka vampire facial) are great options for reducing scarring. Micro-needling utilizes micro-punctures in the skin that stimulate wound healing, producing new collagen and elastin.

Special topicals like stem cells and growth factors can be infused into the skin to help regenerate new skin and reduce scarring. This is also one of the safest scar-reducing treatments on the market. The risks involved with micro-needling are minimal compared to more invasive laser resurfacing and medical-peel treatments. Micro-needling is also safe for darker skin tones which have limited options for acne-scar reduction treatments.

PRP is the practice of injecting your own spun-down blood plasma into your skin to promote the production of collagen and elastin to reduce scarring. It often is administered with micro-needling.

Multiple treatments are necessary to see improvement because collagen production takes time. Treatments are usually spaced four to six weeks apart, and you should begin to see a difference in a few months.

How many treatments will you need? Every person is different. Every case is different. Expect to complete at least five or six treatments, and if you have severe acne scarring, the number of potential treatments is limitless. It all depends on the results you want and what your budget allows.

If cost and downtime are not an issue and you are light in skin color, laser resurfacing might be more cost-effective in the long-run, and you can do it in addition to micro-needling. If you are darker skinned or do not want serious downtime, then micro-needling is the best option to soften and smooth the appearance of scars. Micro-needling requires topical numbing cream and is tolerable, but unpleasant.

NOTE: If numbing cream is not offered for micro-needling, then it is not a clinical treatment and you should find another practitioner. It will be the equivalent of a home-care device, which will be even more costly and nowhere near as effective at reducing your acne scarring.

Downtime for micro-needling is typically a day or two. You can wear foundation 24 hours after treatment, which is another great advantage of this option. Micro-needling or at-home needling devices are not intended for individuals with active acne. The amount of inflammation and minor trauma caused by the micro-needling is enough to instigate an acne breakout, which will not be worth it. Creating the potential for more scarring is counterproductive. Get your acne under control first.

DERMAL FILLERS

Dermal fillers are phenomenal for "ice-pick" scars and atopic (thin, flat or depressed) scars. They replace volume under the skin where it has been lost. Most fillers are hyaluronic-based and are a natural substance found in the body. Results are immediate, and you may require a touch-up treatment for ideal results because it is better to under treat (not enough filler) than over treat (too much filler) acne scars. You don't want to wind up with a mound versus a divot on your skin. (The results of dermal fillers last up to a year.)

My Recommendation: Complete a series of chemical peels, micro-needling or laser resurfacing before opting for dermal fillers to reduce your acne scars. These treatments will help build collagen and possibly eliminate the need for fillers.

LASER RESURFACING

The different technologies and brand names can make the concept of laser resurfacing difficult to understand. There is non-ablative laser resurfacing such as fractional and pulsed dye. These do not remove layers of skin, but rather penetrate through the skin in an attempt to stimulate new collagen production from underneath with about seven to ten days of downtime, depending on the strength and depth of the laser.

Ablative lasers like Erbium, Yag and CO_2 remove layers of skin from the scars' surface, and the heat from the laser helps to tighten the skin and smooth out the scar. Ablative lasers can be very effective in reducing the appearance of scarring. However, it can be very costly, as much as thousands, and the downtime can be significant. Whatever the doctor says your downtime will be, double it. I recommend laser treatments only for individuals who are no longer experiencing acne.

Laser resurfacing carries more risk and is not intended for skin of color (regardless of what you are told). Even light skins of color should be very skeptical of any laser treatments because of their potential to cause hyperpigmentation. The light plus heat can induce inflammation that can also cause a breakout. The thick occlusive creams used to protect your skin's barrier during the healing process can also cause a breakout. Unless your scars are severe, do not start with lasers. This is your last option – not first.

DERMABRASION/MICRODERMABRASION

Dermabrasion is a surgical procedure where a rotary abrasive instrument is utilized to "sand down" the scar for a smoother appearance. The results with dermabrasion can be successful provided you can find a qualified doctor. The downtime for dermabrasion is a minimum of two weeks.

Microdermabrasion, the "watered-down" version of dermabrasion, will not smooth out scars permanently. Scarring may seem to have been reduced because when the dead skin is removed, the scar appears less noticeable. I use microdermabrasion in my acne treatments as an ancillary treatment to peels and micro-needling because it enhances the results, but it is superficial and typically does not permanently diminish the scar.

TRICHLOROACETIC ACID CROSS

Trichloroacetic Acid (TCA) Cross uses a high percentage of TCA inside the scar that stimulates collagen production and causes the scar to lift up and close in on itself. The downtime is localized to the size of the scar. This treatment can be hit or miss in terms of results.

SCAR EXCISION OR PUNCH EXCISION

Scar Excision/Punch Excision is a surgical method that uses a scalpel or punch to remove the scar and stitch the skin edges together for a less noticeable scar. This method is reserved for deep scarring, as the scar it leaves behind obviously needs to be smaller than the original acne scar itself.

CONCLUSION

Acne is on the rise globally, and according to conventional medicine, there is no cure. However, just because standard westernized medicine does not know or have the cure does not mean there is no cure for acne. With all the advancements in modern medicine, there are still so many things we do not know or fully understand about the human body.

The increase in acne is due to our food supply, if you can call it that. It has been grossly altered to barely resemble food, and the mass production of harmful chemicals over the last 50 years have been added to virtually everything we eat, buy, sit on, clean with and wear. This is causing your acne, damaging your health in a multitude of ways and prematurely aging you.

Pharmaceutical companies want our doctors and the public to believe they need some pill to "cure" or "control" whatever condition or disease they have been diagnosed with. These same companies want you to believe changing your diet and lifestyle habits will not eliminate the need for prescription medication.

There is big money being invested in the marketing of foods, prescription medications and cosmetics, which is why we are being inundated with advertising that essentially brainwashes us and creates false common knowledge about our eating, lifestyle and spending habits.

The answer is making better choices in what we put in and around our bodies. You can be sure that following what I have laid out will (at the very least) make your acne better than it was and, in most cases, cure it entirely. It will not make your acne condition worse, jeopardize your health or cause unwanted side effects. There is no risk in eating an organic plant-based diet, using non-toxic cosmetics and cleaning products, getting better rest and reducing exposure to unnecessary stressors. Your overall health will improve drastically and help you maintain beautiful skin.

I tell my clients it may be easier to start with one step at a time, like reducing or eliminating dairy for starters. Start replacing all of your cleaning and cosmetic products one-by-one with "greener" alternatives to stop compounding the toxic burden on your body. Drink one cup of organic coffee per day versus two triple-pump sugar lattes. The point is to get started, maybe with the easy stuff first.

Many people gasp and say, "What is left to eat?" I remind them what I originally stated, "You can cure your acne, but you won't like my answer!" All jokes aside, there are plenty of great tasting healthy foods out there, but you are going to have to make some changes and re-train your taste buds.

Real food actually tastes better and is more satisfying once your body has had a chance to get acclimated to the transition. Believe it or not, you will eventually start craving healthful foods and stop desiring the crappy ones. Even better, more farm-to-table-style restaurants are opening up everywhere offering tasty plant-based dishes with gluten free, dairy free, and non-GMO choices. *Heck, they even have Kombucha on tap now!*

Let me also clarify that in the majority of cases, following these steps will clear acne, but it does not mean you will never again experience another pimple. Acne is not having a few pimples from time to time. Your success is going to depend on how serious you are in curing your acne. It is not going to be as easy as taking a pill or buying products and treatments, because if that alone worked, there would be no demand for me to write this book.

How fast your acne heals depends on how fast you implement these recommendations and how disciplined you are at following them. It also takes time to heal your gut from all the assaults it has had to endure for many years. This will take some patience. Following these steps may seem overwhelming, but it is totally possible. I see it happen all the time. Now that you are clear, I know that you can do it!

Be sure to check out the Additional Resources for books you might like, recommended products, handy checklists and more.

Next Steps

---

1. If you got value from this book, please leave a review on Amazon.

2. Be sure to sign up for my
   Celebrity Skincare Newsletter at:
   www.CelebritySkinScottsdale.com/gettingclear
   where you'll receive monthly tips and special
   promotions for beautiful, healthy skin.

Additional Resources

WHAT IS...

ENVIRONMENTAL WORKING GROUP?

EWG is a non-partisan organization designed to help you protect your health by providing information about toxins in your environment that affect children's health, toxics, consumer products, energy, farming, food and water. For more information, visit **www.ewg.org.**

THE CELIAC DISEASE FOUNDATION?

The Celiac Disease Foundation drives diagnosis, treatment and a cure to improve the quality of life for all people affected by celiac disease and non-celiac gluten or wheat sensitivity. For a complete list of code words for gluten, visit **www.celiac.org**.

KIDS WITH FOOD ALLERGIES?

Kids with Food Allergies (KFA) is an organization that offers free tools, educational materials, webinars, videos and other resources to help families keep children (and adults) safe and healthy. For more information, visit **www.kidswithfoodallergies.org.**

SUGAR SCIENCE?

Sugar Science, *The Unsweetened Truth* is designed as an authoritative source for the scientific evidence about sugar and its impact on health. For a complete list of sugar names and scary facts, visit **www.sugarscience.ucsf.edu.**

WEBMD.COM?

Web MD is a medical team that helps to provide valuable and credible health information, tools for managing your health, and support to those who seek information. For up-to-date, accurate medical information, visit **www.webmd.com.**

DRUGS.COM?

This website is a well-trusted Internet resource presenting independent, objective, comprehensive and up-to-date information for drug and related health information. For a list of drugs, their side effects and potential interactions with other types of medications, supplements or food, visit **www.drugs.com.**

THE ORGANIC CONSUMERS ASSOCIATION?

The Organic Consumers Association is an online non-profit public-interest organization campaigning for health, justice and sustainability. The OCA deals with crucial issues of food safety, industrial agriculture, genetic engineering, children's health, corporate accountability, Fair Trade, environmental sustainability and other key topics.

OCA is a great resource for information regarding organic standards, cooking organic, toxic products/cosmetics in your home and which mainstream commercial corporations and government agencies are not being honest about what they are feeding or telling you. For more information, visit **www.organicconsumers.org.**

MORE ABOUT...

LEAKY GUT

- Information on leaky gut – **www.drweil.com** and **www.draxe.com**
- Book- Eat Dirt by Dr. Josh Axe - **www.draxe.com**
- Book – Grain Brain by David Perlmutter, M.D. – **www.drperlmutter.com**

DIET

- Paleo Diet Information and Guidelines – **www.paleoleap.com**

- Paleo vs. Vegan Diet – The Pros and Cons – **www.draxe.com**
- Anti-Inflammatory Diet – **www.drweil.com**
- The WHOLE30™ Diet – **www.whole30.com**
- The Gaps Diet – **www.gapsdiet.com**
- Intermittent Fasting – **www.healthline.com**
- Book – *The Paleo Approach* by Sarah Ballantyne, PhD – **www.thepaleomom.com**
- Book – *Dr. Kellyann's Bone Broth Cookbook* by Dr. Kellyann – **www.drkellyann.com**
- Book – *Eat Dirt* by Dr. Josh Axe – **www.draxe.com**
- Documentary – Food Matters (Netflix)
- Documentary – Fed Up (Netflix)
- Documentary – Cowspiracy: The Sustainability Secret (Netflix)
- Documentary – Forks over Knives (Netflix)
- Documentary – Fat, Sick and Nearly Dead (Netflix)
- Documentary – Gut Reaction (Top Documentary Films)
- Documentary – Beyond Food

DRINKING WATER

For information on safe drinking water, how to reduce your exposure to common drinking-water pollutants, which types of water are best to drink (spring, tap, alkaline), which bottled water brands and water-filtration systems are better, visit **www.ewg.org**

- Bottled water – Evian, Mountain Valley Spring Water (in glass instead of plastic and comes in 5-gallon jugs too), Hawaiian Water, Ice Age water, Arrowhead, Volvic and Poland are some good brands.
- Home-water-filtration system – Revitalizer made by Pure Effect Advanced Filtration.
- Water filtration for showerheads – Aqua Bliss
- Documentary – Secret of Water; Discover the Language of Life

SUPPLEMENTS

Good quality brands for supplemental nutrition: Thorn, Vital Nutrients, Garden of Life, Douglas Labs, Jarrows, New Chapter, Enzymatic Therapy, Pure Encapsulations, Nordic Naturals and New Life.

Where can you buy quality supplements? Many of your local health-food grocery stores carry good-quality supplements. Avoid purchasing supplements from vitamin stores that only carry their brands. You can also visit www.amazon.com.

STRESS

Guided Meditation – Deepak Choprah and Oprah Winfrey offer 20 minute, downloadable guided-meditation programs or various subjects specifically designed to make meditation easy and effective. For more information, visit **www.chopracentermeditation.com.**

MORE ABOUT SLEEP

The National Sleep Foundation offers information on sleep topics, disorders and where to find help. For more information, visit **www.sleepfoundation.org**

For information on beauty sleep, visit **www.Webmd.com**

HORMONES

Hormone Health Network is an international resource center on hormones as they relate to your health, diseases and conditions. For more information on hormones, visit **www.hormone.org**.

Information on the link between diet and hormone levels, visit **www.mercola.com**

- Book – *It's Your Hormones* by Geoffrey Redmond, M.D. – **www.amazon.com**

TOXINS

For more information on toxic chemicals in our food and personal and home-care products, visit **www.ewg.org**

- Book – *TOX-SICK: From Toxic to Not Sick* by Suzanne Somers- **www.suzannesomers.com**

Documentary – The Human Experiment (Netflix). Shocking reality of untested chemicals in our everyday products.

- Coffee Enemas. For more information about how to

do coffee enemas and where to purchase supplies, visit
www.gerson.org

- FAR Infrared Saunas – For more information on where
  to purchase them, visit **www.therasage.com**

NON-TOXIC HOME AND PERSONAL CARE PRODUCTS

The following list of home-care products are safer alternatives
for use in your home:

- E-Cover, Seventh Generation, Mrs. Meyer's, EO,
  EcoSmart, Natural Value and Purelight

These brands offer safer laundry detergents, hand and dish
soaps, cleaning products, plastic bags, sandwhich bags, cups,
plates, paper towels, tissues, sponges, bath products, baby
products, pet care, bug repellants, home pest control and
garden care.

COSMETICS

The following list of cosmetics are safer alternatives to use on
your skin and body:

- Neuma, Davines, Jane Iredale, Advanced Mineral
  Makeup, Vapour Organic Beauty, Weleda, Herban
  Cowboy, Osmia & Seaweed Bath Co., Schwarzkopf
  Essensity, Rhonda Allison, and Desert Essence.

These brands offer safer shampoos, conditioners, hair-styling products, permanent hair colors/dyes, body lotions/washes, cosmetics, foundations, deodorants, toothpastes, and skin-care products.

For a list of pore-clogging ingredients in beauty supplies, visit **www.facerealityacneclinic.com**

ACNE CHECKLIST

Want to get clear? Here's a handy checklist to follow for better skin:

- ☐ Eliminate dairy/limit dairy
- ☐ Limit/eliminate all grains
- ☐ Eliminate gluten
- ☐ Limit/eliminate caffeine
- ☐ Limit/eliminate alcohol
- ☐ Limit/eliminate vegetable oils/Omega-6 oils
- ☐ Complete a candida and liver cleanse
- ☐ Incorporate bone broth
- ☐ Take supplements
- ☐ Eliminate dehydration both internally and topically
- ☐ Detox your home and body from harmful toxins
- ☐ Reduce stress
- ☐ Practice good sleep
- ☐ Get a naturopathic doctor if you can afford one
- ☐ Get clinical facials and skin-care products
- ☐ Get a dermatologist (if necessary)

MEDICAL TESTING LIST

You may want to test for these to make sure there aren't any underlying conditions that could be exacerbating your skin problems:

- ☐ Comprehensive Hormone Panel Test including-
  - ☐ Estrogen
  - ☐ Estradiol
  - ☐ Estrone
  - ☐ DHT
  - ☐ Testosterone
  - ☐ SHBG
  - ☐ DHEA
  - ☐ Progesterone
  - ☐ Cortisol
- ☐ Thyroid
  - ☐ TSH
  - ☐ T3
  - ☐ T4
- ☐ Food Allergy Test
- ☐ Gluten-Sensitivity Test
- ☐ CBC and CMP Test
- ☐ A1C or Fasting Insulin Test
- ☐ Candida Test
- ☐ Vitamin D Test